Forge Your Inner Armor

Strengthen Your Brain-Body Connections to Perform at Your Potential

Dr. Timothy Royer
with Gregory Smith

Inner Armor Media

Copyright © 2023 Timothy Royer
All rights reserved.
ISBN: 9798386675356

To our Creator, who made us in his image and gave us brains that can see and feel, think and choose, move and make, imagine and create. We are fearfully and wonderfully made.

CONTENTS

	Acknowledgments	i
1	Performance Matters	1
2	You Are a Miracle	7
3	System of Systems	14
4	Command and Control	23
5	Prime Directive	31
6	Response and Resilience	37
7	Measuring the Mind	44
8	Frequency and Focus	52
9	Coherent Power	60
10	Precise Coordination	67
11	Stress Loading	75
12	Training and Technology	85
13	Inner Armor	92
	About the Authors	99

ACKNOWLEDGMENTS

Sir Isaac Newton, who discovered the laws of motion and gravity, and (oh, by the way) invented calculus, refused to take credit for his accomplishments. He said, "If I have seen further, it is by standing on the shoulders of giants."

That's all that I, and my team at Royer Neuroscience and Inner Armor, have done. We are integrators who apply the insights and inventions of giants so that everyone, from ordinary people to professional athletes, might live better, more resilient lives. And so it's only fitting to acknowledge some of those giants.

First are the pioneers in neuroscience and psychology who reframed our understanding of the brain-body connection. Ivan Pavlov (1849-1936), a Russian neurologist, psychologist, and physiologist, discovered the principles of classical conditioning through his experiments with dogs. B.F. Skinner (1904-1990), an American psychologist, innovated the use of operant or instrumental conditioning to strengthen behavior. Hans

Selye (1907-1982) was a Hungarian-Canadian endocrinologist who changed our understanding of how environments and situations create biological responses and first used the word "stress" to describe this effect. Robert Sapolsky is an American neuroendocrinology researcher that has made invaluable contributions to understanding how stress contributes to disease. Standing on their shoulders, we are learning to use neurophysiological training to improve human performance, reduce destructive stress, and avoid degenerative disease.

Second are the pioneers in biofeedback technology. Just as a pilot uses an altimeter and airspeed indicator to fly the plane better, their inventions allow us to perform better by monitoring our brains and bodies in real time. Of particular note is the German physiologist Hans Berger (1873–1941), who developed the first electroencephalography (EEG) monitor in 1924. Before that, the brain seemed even more mysterious because we could not "see" or measure the electrical signals racing through our neural networks. And it was Barry Sterman, whose story we tell in chapter 8, that combined EEG technology with operant conditioning techniques to identify and optimize brainwave frequencies to boost resilience. Standing on their shoulders, we can understand how our brain is performing and train it to perform better.

Finally, we must recognize the pioneers of the personal computer revolution. Almost everyone has heard of Bill Gates, Steve Jobs, and Steve Wozniak, but they stood on the shoulders of giants before them, and others have built on their work. This revolution has changed the world. Although it has brought its share of negative consequences for human health and performance, it has also given Royer Neuroscience and Inner Armor the tools to apply the best principles of neuroscience and biofeedback to build better lives. Standing on their shoulders, we can offer ordinary people practical training in everyday life.

Progress continues, and every year there are more discoveries and inventions. My team and I will continue to innovate how we integrate and apply the best of what science and technology offer to help you become dynamically resilient and perform at your potential.

Dr. Timothy Royer

CHAPTER 1
PERFORMANCE MATTERS

Because you are a fusion of mind and body, the efficiency and effectiveness of that connection determine your performance.

Potential encourages and effort inspires. But in the end, performance matters.

That's easier to see in athletics because sports keep scores and statistics. We admire players who give it everything they've got, but the win goes to those who put the most points on the board. Those are the players who converted their potential and effort into performance on the field.

The same can be said for the classroom, the boardroom, or the control room. Students, business people, and operators of everything from power plants to submarines and manufacturing lines have to perform. Learning, earning, or managing successfully depends on catalyzing potential and effort to solve problems and produce results.

But this is true even in less obvious arenas. Every day, families have to get up, get moving, and get things done. We have to get to where we need to be, on time, with our materials in hand and our homework completed. Children need to be fed and clothed, loved and disciplined. Moms and dads must perform even when they are tired, stressed, and unmotivated. Dogs need walking, homes need maintenance, and bills need paying.

In all that we try to do, getting it done, and done well, matters. Good intentions are great, but actions speak louder than words. If you want to be successful at anything—relationships, work, or sports—a pretty reliable formula is to be where you're supposed to be, when you're supposed to be there, doing what you're supposed to do, as well as you're capable of doing it. Yes, someone else might get there earlier and do it better, but if you get the most out of your potential and effort, then you've succeeded.

Most of us know (but don't want to admit) that we often fall short of our potential and don't get the best results from our efforts. We look back at the day, or the project, or the game and realize that we were capable of more. We could have and should have performed better than we did.

So we feel guilty and tell ourselves that we'll try harder next time. Sometimes that works. Sometimes we focus more and lean deeper into the next challenge, and we pull it off.

But only sometimes. Our outcomes could be better. Even with plenty of preparation and the best of intentions, even when we have a good practice or study session, our plans don't always translate into reliable performances.

Why?

Because what we might call the "performance equation" contains more variables than just *potential* and *effort*. Variables like *command, control,* and *action*. For better or worse, potential and effort are multiplied by your ability to command and control your body and translate your will into actions.

Athletics is, by definition, a matter of physical performance. And many of us who aren't athletically gifted figured out when we were in school that we'd never succeed in sports and instead chose less physically demanding work or hobbies.

But here's the thing: almost everything we must do must be done in the physical world. Waking up in the morning doesn't take much physical effort. But getting up, making your bed, and starting the day right are tangible actions that take physical effort and discipline. Going to school, catching a flight, feeding your baby, making a presentation, making home repairs, grading papers, and even sitting at your keyboard writing a book; all of these involve translating your mental will into tangible physical actions within the real world. And that requires commanding and controlling your body to carry out your decisions and plans.

This transfer of will into action is where so much of your performance breaks down. Your alarm goes off, but you don't get up and make the bed. You scroll your social media over coffee and lose track of time. You can't find your keys, so you're late getting out the door. You try to juggle too many things while talking on the phone and spill your coffee as you set up your work area or board a plane. Your eyes hurt from staring at the computer screen, your back aches, and your head pounds from stress as the deadline nears. Your hands shake as you lie under the sink, trying to get the screws into the holes while repairing the garbage disposal. You get so nervous before the meeting that you fumble your answers to the boss' questions. You're so exhausted that you almost fall asleep behind the wheel driving home. By the end of the day, you're so burnt out that you don't play with your kids, talk to your spouse, or call your mother. The stress makes you self-medicate with alcohol or cannabis, Netflix or video games.

Anything worth doing requires really doing something in the real world. You may not catch passes in the NFL or fly a fighter jet, but success takes more than bright ideas and a positive attitude.

Even winning video games involves translating thought into bodily action, and I can prove it: play against a 13-year-old. I know actual NFL players that get destroyed in NFL video games by some kid, even when the real-life player is playing his virtual self in the game. How can that be? The real-life player knows more about football, and his virtual self's skills, than the kid ever will. But knowledge and motivation aren't enough. Winning the video game requires lightning-quick reflexes and muscle memory of the game controller. No matter how quick the real-life player is on the real-life field, his neural pathways, visual processing speed, reflexes, and mastery of the game controller are no match for the kid's.

My point is that much of life depends upon a close connection between the mind and body. Your success in almost any endeavor is determined by how well you can command and control your body to perform. But your mind-body connection isn't always as tight or reliable as you'd like it to be. Anyone who's ever tried to play golf has discovered that you can't always make your body do what you want it to when you want it to.

Why?

Because you are a fusion of mind and body, the efficiency and effectiveness of that connection determine your performance. Your will has to be translated into action. Just because you are capable of something, and because you want it badly and try very hard to do it, doesn't mean that your body will respond the way you want it to. The feedback loops between your body and brain are only sometimes accurate. Your organs and muscles don't always respond when you tell them to in the way you want them to. If there's a lot of noise in the system, then much of your effort gets wasted, and too much of your potential is unmet. Your spirit might be willing, but far too often, the flesh is weak.

Physical or psychological training can improve aspects of human performance. But they leave out a hidden element that's upstream, influencing our physical and psychological condition. It operates autonomously and unconsciously. But more than anything else, it determines how effectively and consistently you can translate your intentions into actions. That hidden performance driver is what this book is all about.

Would you like to gain greater command and control of your body and transfer that into more effective action? Then read on.

CHAPTER 2
YOU ARE A MIRACLE

You are a miracle, and your brain is the most dazzling part of it. Even on your worst day, your brain is still the most amazing thing in the universe.

When I was young, I learned that helping people to build better lives begins with genuinely understanding their core needs and then targeting solutions to meet them. I learned that in Africa, of all places.

The summer after I graduated from high school, I took a turn that would change my life. My father was a college football coach, and I grew up around many famous college and professional athletes. After my dad died in a plane crash, my mother married a chaplain to several professional sports teams. I was planning on attending the United States Naval Academy in the fall (my dad's friend, legendary Notre Dame football coach Lou Holtz, wrote my Academy recommendation). But a few weeks before I was supposed to show up in Annapolis, I decided that my heart wasn't in it. All of a sudden, I had no idea what I wanted to do, but I knew it wasn't college and sports.

My stepfather was president of a mission organization building a hospital in the West African nation of Togo. He saw me struggling to figure out the world and my place in it, so he suggested I take some time to see what I could learn there. I was eighteen and had never been out of the USA before, but my folks put me on a plane and sent me to this unfamiliar place where I knew no one.

When I got there, I learned to work with my hands: construction, carpentry, welding—I did anything that needed to be done. I learned how to turn mahogany and teak trees into two-by-fours with a chainsaw and a planer. I learned to work outside under the sun in the African countryside. And over the months, where the road ended far out in the bush a long way from town, we built a hospital.

That's when and where I realized that I wanted to help people. I saw how much of the world lives, how so many people live with so few resources, and how significant their challenges are. We were always short-staffed, and everyone had to pitch in to do everything, so I got to assist in the hospital. Here I found my calling. I discovered that I was supposed to help people feeling overwhelmed by life to break down their problems into manageable pieces. If I could do that and then help them solve those smaller, more fundamental problems, I could help them build a better future for themselves.

I realized that I needed to go home and get an education. I ended up at Cedarville University, a small liberal arts college outside Dayton, Ohio. On my first day there, I met Amy, who would eventually become my wife of 34 years. She, too, had grown up building hospitals in the developing world; her family had been medical missionaries in Bangladesh. Surprisingly, it turned out that her folks knew my stepdad. We both knew God had made us life partners with the same mission.

We got married in college. I graduated with a degree in psychology, Amy in nursing. We ended up in Atlanta, where she worked as a pediatric bone marrow transplant nurse, and I worked on my doctorate. By the time I finished, Amy was expecting, and I found an internship at a psychiatric hospital in Michigan.

In 1994, I got an opportunity to make a real difference. I was asked to start, from scratch, a pediatric psychology and psychiatry division at DeVos Children's Hospital in Grand Rapids, Michigan. In our first year, we saw 150 kids. By the time I left, it was over 4,000 per year. As the division chief, my staff and I dealt with the behavioral needs of children in every way imaginable, from supporting kids undergoing surgery to counseling them in ICU after suicide attempts. But the most significant part of what we did—and what started me down the path of writing this book—was neuropsychological testing. We examined children with every possible symptom, searching for the underlying causes. We dealt with conditions as ordinary as learning difficulties and unusual as brain tumors. We saw a lot of kids with Attention Deficit Hyperactivity Disorder (ADHD) because their numbers were snowballing during the 1990s and early 2000s. Instead of just prescribing drugs, I wanted to understand why. What was causing this apparent epidemic? I knew that unless we figured that out, we could never hope to help these children build better lives.

I wanted more accurate, data-driven diagnostic tools to identify what was actually causing ADHD and other behavioral disorders. It was clear that these symptoms originated in the brain and nervous system. Psychoanalysis, or "talking therapy," couldn't explain, much less fix, them. Drugs didn't work. What could, exactly?

Eventually, I left the hospital to open a private practice focused on helping people to regulate their autonomic nervous system (ANS). I then co-founded a company with Dr. Brad Oostindie called Hope139, dedicated to using neuroscience to help people strengthen their brains and ANS. Since then, my work has developed into utilizing neuroscience technology to help anyone, including athletes and executives, perform more consistently at their potential by gaining more control over their mind-body connection.

As a teenager building that hospital in Africa, I learned that building better lives requires rolling up our sleeves and doing the sometimes challenging work of understanding what needs to be done, gathering the right resources, and patiently solving the actual problems. Compassion requires a genuine understanding of people's problems and what they need to build better lives. Particular problems require particular solutions. And the specific problem I feel compelled to address is the abuse, misuse, and neglect of the mind-body connection.

The nexus of this connection is the brain.

Your brain is one of the most stunningly complex and surprisingly beautiful things in all the universe. Ironically, only a human brain could judge something as stunning and beautiful and compose that sentence.

You are one of the most amazing parts of this vast and complex universe. One or two hundred pounds of biological matter that can think and feel, compose and create, build and travel, learn and teach. You are not just quantitatively better at all these things than other animals; you are qualitatively different. And the most incredible part of your fantastic body is your brain. It is, perhaps, the greatest of God's creations.

Because it drives all of your activity, your brain consumes an enormous amount of your body's energy. It amounts to about 2% of your total body weight—nearly half the weight of your skin—but it uses 20% of your body's blood and oxygen. When your body is at rest, your brain burns 20% of your calories, but it is marvelously efficient in using that energy. A typical adult human brain runs on about twelve watts of power. Compare that to the sixty-watt light bulb in your bedside lamp or the eighty watts my laptop uses while I write this paragraph. But my computer only recorded the words that my brain imagined and composed. And while the smartest supercomputers greedily consume hundreds of thousands of watts on distributed server networks, they are created and controlled by human brains humming along, using less power than a small flashlight.

Not impressed yet? The human brain has about a hundred billion neurons, roughly the same as the number of stars in our galaxy. They are fed by over 400 miles of blood vessels. But each of those neurons has ten thousand (or more) synapses, which can combine with all the synapses around them in a nearly infinite combination of neural pathways. Those dozen watts of electricity race through those pathways at almost two hundred miles per hour. Hundreds of billions of neurons with hundreds of trillions of connections and pathways. For all intents and purposes, your brain is infinitely complex. As the poet Emily Dickinson put it,

> *The brain is wider than the sky,*
> *For, put them side by side,*
> *The one the other will include*
> *With ease, and you beside.*

> *The brain is deeper than the sea,*

For, hold them, blue to blue,
The one the other will absorb,
As sponges, buckets do.

The brain is just the weight of God,
For, lift them, pound for pound
And they will differ, if they do,
As syllable from sound.

Your brain is deeper than the sea and bears the weight of God. Wow! You are a miracle, and your brain is the most dazzling part of it. Even on your worst day, your brain is still the most amazing thing in the universe. So, why would you not treat your brain with all the reverence it deserves?

Don't take your brain-body connection for granted. Too often, we damage our brains with unhealthy lifestyles, environments, and substances. Then we wonder why we can't perform consistently near our potential. We don't understand why we are growing less healthy and happy, so we look for simplistic explanations and convenient solutions that solve nothing, and consequently, our performance never really improves.

But there is hope because much of what ails us can be understood and addressed through documentable, quantifiable biology and neuroscience.

CHAPTER 3
SYSTEM OF SYSTEMS

Performing consistently at or near your potential requires aggregate coordination. And this is the problem with so many performance plans and training systems: they don't look at the critical interactions between the body's systems.

You are a system of systems.

In other words, your body is a collection of billions of distinct cells, tissues, organs, and systems, but all of these collaborate, forming a "meta-system." And that meta-system is you, a human person in all of your incredible complexity.

Smaller units organize into larger structures. So, thousands or millions of specialized cells collectively form tissues. Specialized tissues are layered to create organs. And groups of organs, some spread far apart throughout the body, work together as coordinated systems to perform complex functions.

There are various ways that these complicated structures can be labeled and numbered, but most often, the human body is described as being composed of eleven major systems. Each system, of course, consists of particular organs, tissues, and cells that communicate and coordinate with each other across the various parts of the body. The systems are distinct but interwoven and interdependent. If one is seriously compromised, the others cannot easily take up the slack.

Let's begin by quickly reviewing these major systems, and then we'll talk about what holds them together and keeps them acting in concert so that you can do everything you do.

Skeletal System. Without your bones, you'd lie there like a jellyfish on the beach. But the skeletal system is not just girders and struts that keep you upright. This system has complex tissues that grow, adapt, and heal. The interior of your bones, the soft spongy marrow, is an incredible cell factory, generating stem cells that form into specialized cells. For example, 95% of the body's red blood cells, which carry oxygen between the respiratory, cardiovascular, and muscular systems, are created in the center of your bones, as are the white blood cells that your immune system uses to fight infection, injury, and illness.

Muscular System. Your muscles enable you to move and perform many other functions you don't think about. For example, they hold you together. Your muscles keep you standing without your organs falling out of the front of your abdomen. They let you do everything from eating and swallowing to focusing your eyes or urinating. Your muscles move when your nervous system tells them to, fueled by oxygen ($O2$) and generating carbon dioxide ($CO2$) as waste. They rely upon the skeletal system to create red blood cells that the respiratory system loads oxygen into like microscopic delivery trucks. The circulatory system transports those trucks to the muscles, where they unload their cargo and then carry away the carbon dioxide and other wastes.

Endocrine System. Spread throughout your body are specialized organs called glands. Among them are the pituitary, thyroid, adrenal, pancreas, ovaries (in women), and testes (in men). These glands release specialized chemicals called hormones, which regulate most of the processes in your body. Glands are like fuel injectors; the hormones they release carry instructions to the organs in other systems to respond in preprogrammed ways. The variety, sequence, and timing of hormones spraying into your bloodstream regulate everything from your metabolism to your moods, growth and sleep, blood pressure, energy level, and more. If this system gets imbalanced, it can cause a cascade of health effects.

Cardiovascular System. Your heart is the pump, and your blood vessels are the highways that cells, hormones, and other compounds move along to get everything in your body to where it needs to be. It works with the respiratory system to send oxygen to the muscles and bring carbon dioxide back from them, nutrition out of the digestive system, and toxins into the urinary system. It carries white blood cells to fight disease and hormones to activate and deactivate processes throughout the body. Near the skin, your blood vessels expand and contract to help regulate your body temperature according to the nervous system's instructions.

Lymphatic System. There is another system of specialized tissues, vessels, and organs spread throughout your body, which creates and transports a fluid called lymph into and out of your bloodstream. This lymphatic fluid is a watery and colorless plasma. It maintains your blood volume (and thus blood pressure) and carries all sorts of compounds and cells: proteins, minerals, fats, nutrients, and white blood cells. But it also carries away dead and damaged cells, including cancer cells. Your lymph nodes are little bean-shaped glands that secrete and cleanse the lymphatic fluid. They are connected by lymph ducts, which have off-ramps into the bloodstream.

Respiratory System. This system consists of more than just your lungs. In addition to bringing oxygen into your body and expelling carbon dioxide, it allows you to talk and smell and adjusts body temperature by warming and moisturizing the air coming into your core. The system involves your mouth, nose, sinuses, and the entire airway into your chest. It also includes your diaphragm, the muscles that move to force air into and out of your lungs. At the microscopic level, your lungs have structures called alveoli. This is where oxygen is exchanged for carbon dioxide, the fuel and exhaust of your body's engine.

Digestive System. Your digestive system breaks down food into building materials for cells and tissues, fuel for energy, and removes waste. But this system, running from your mouth to your anus, is an entire ecosystem composed of subsystems that are dynamically interdependent on other body systems and coordinated by a complex set of signals sent through nerves and hormones. It is also a point of interface with the outside world and, thus, a potential source of contamination and infection that must be countered through feedback loops with other systems.

Urinary System. Your blood circulates, carrying life-giving cargo (oxygen, hormones, nutrients, etc.) to cells and tissues throughout the body. When it delivers that cargo, it picks up the trash: chemical waste from cellular processes, toxins, etc. If these build up in tissues or the bloodstream, you'll get seriously ill and eventually die. So, the blood passes through filters located in organs called kidneys. These separate the harmful compounds from the helpful ones and remove the bad stuff by manufacturing urine, which passes out of the body. This process is almost entirely involuntary and unconscious, except when your bladder tells your brain it needs to be emptied. But this signal can be interrupted or accelerated by other processes, including stress.

Reproductive System. Living creatures are programmed with a biological imperative to ensure the survival of the species by passing on their genetic material on to another generation. The reproductive system serves this powerful instinct. But the other systems of the body are dynamically connected with it. Powerful signals, hormonal balances, growth, and metabolic cycles are sent and received by the reproductive system. In various ways, it can influence our ability to perform at our potential at any particular time.

Integumentary System. This is the outermost layer of your body, including your skin and its appendages (hair, nails, etc.). It forms a physical barrier between the outside world and your interior bones, tissues, and organs. But it's not a mere shell or covering. It has layers of semi-permeable tissues that maintain water balance, regulates temperature, and excrete wastes. It's also loaded with sensory receptor cells that detect pressure, pain, taste, and temperature.

Nervous System. As we saw in the last chapter, this complex system runs through your body like the electrical system in an airplane or building. It is subdivided into the central nervous system (your brain and spinal column) and your peripheral nervous system (PNS), which runs out to the rest of your body. Your PNS is further subdivided into the somatic (or voluntary) nervous system (SNS) and the autonomic nervous system (ANS). We're going to be talking extensively about the nervous system in the next chapter because it is the system that commands, controls, and coordinates all the other systems.

As you can see, bodily functions span multiple systems and require synchronization. Everything, from unconscious processes like growth to complex tasks like playing the piano or catching footballs, involves an intricate dance of organs and systems controlling specialized cells and tissues using electrical and chemical signals.

These systems are vulnerable to injury and illness and can (and should be) strengthened. Improving systems will increase our potential to perform life's complex demands and tasks.

But when it comes to improvement or training, we tend to consider systems in isolation from the whole. For example, one school of thought might emphasize strength training, building up the skeletal and muscular systems for health and performance. Another school of thought will emphasize gut health, hormones, cardiovascular fitness, diet, and weight. These are undeniably helpful, and improving any system will enhance our general health and raise our performance potential.

But these specific approaches don't always address the totality of our performance, what it takes to achieve our potential consistently, on demand at any given moment. Consider an athlete who lifts weights, eats right, has a low pulse rate, manages her gut health, and pays attention to her body's chemical and hormonal balances. She is already far ahead of where she would be without doing those things, and she has raised her capacity to perform her sport and the probability of performing well in her next competition. But none of that guarantees that she will play her best.

Why? Because performance depends upon her various systems being calibrated and synchronized. Her muscles must work in concert with her visual processing through the nervous system, but the cardiovascular and respiratory systems need to be coherent to maximize her power. Her endocrine system must release adrenaline and other hormones in the proper sequence and at the right moments. The capillaries near her skin need to contract or expand to manage her body temperature, along with the endocrine system controlling her sweat mechanisms. Her digestive system needs to deliver the proper nutrients and compounds for her muscles to perform, her urinary tract has to filter toxins, and so on. Her performance on the court depends on the strength of the individual systems and how well they work together.

If she is a student-athlete, she also has to study for exams. Again, her eyes, brain, and muscles must work together, visually processing hundreds of pages of material. Her digestive system needs to release energy and nutrients to maintain health throughout exam week. During the exams, her respiratory and cardiovascular systems need to maintain a steady rhythm, sending oxygen to her brain and not forcing her into a panic state in which she can't remember what she's learned. Her systems need to keep psychological stress from causing digestive or urinary stress.

Because you are a system of systems, performing consistently at or near your potential requires aggregate coordination. And this is the problem with so many performance plans and training systems: they don't look at the critical interactions between the body's systems. Because something hidden below the surface commands and controls, regulating and coordinating the systems of systems that is you.

CHAPTER 4
COMMAND AND CONTROL

Your body and mind can only work well together if they are synchronized. And if your ANS is not cooperating with your conscious mind and physical systems, your outcomes will be inconsistent and below your expectations.

Your car has miles of wires running through it, connecting components through switches and relays to instruments and mini-computers. In the same way, your body has a nervous system that receives information from all its parts, processes that data, and sends commands back to control your actions. The nervous system itself is composed of subsystems. Your central nervous system (CNS) is composed of your brain and spinal cord. But your peripheral nervous system (PNS) connects your central nervous system to your sensory organs and skeletal muscles.

This peripheral nervous system is further subdivided into two subsystems. The first is the somatic nervous system. It's also called the voluntary nervous system because you are conscious of it and can voluntarily control it. For example, if your eyes observe that it's starting to rain and you feel the raindrops on your skin, you might decide to put on your raincoat, and you command your muscles to get it out of your pack and pull it on. Or you could choose to head indoors and command yourself to walk home. Or you might decide that the rain is no big deal and command yourself to stay put. Those inputs, decisions, and actions are all functions of the somatic, or voluntary, nervous system.

But that's not all that's happening in your body. Much or even most of what your brain and body do falls below the level of consciousness. Right now, you're breathing without reminding yourself to breathe. Your heart is pumping without you telling it to do so. Your intestinal tract is digesting food, your body is regulating its core temperature, and your glands are injecting chemicals into your bloodstream to perform a hundred different tasks. You're unaware that your brain is monitoring, commanding, and controlling your systems while you read these words. But it is, or you'd die before the end of this chapter. All of this functions autonomously, in the background, without your direct input. And all this autonomous command and control is managed by the autonomic nervous system (sometimes called the involuntary nervous system), which I will often refer to in this book as the ANS.

The ANS is a hidden command and control network regulating your internal organs: your heart, lungs, liver, stomach, intestines, urinary tract, gall bladder, sex organs, pancreas, blood vessels, lymph nodes, etc. And it coordinates those organs to manage much of what takes place "under the hood" in your body. The ANS relegates your blood pressure; how fast your heart beats and your rate of breathing; the constriction of your blood vessels; your body temperature; your digestion; your response to stress; when and how much you sweat; your metabolism and body weight, the percentage of electrolytes in your hydration; how much saliva, sweat, and tears you secrete; when you need to urinate or defecate; your sexual urges and responses. On and on it goes. Your ANS is the hidden operating system that keeps your body operating and determines how well it will perform.

And it is the determining factor for how well you will perform in almost any situation. Because when your conscious mind wants to do anything, it has to get your body's unconscious organs and processes to cooperate. Your ability to command and control your body's actions depends upon the strength of that mind-body connection.

Even if you have fantastic innate physical abilities and well-developed skills and are highly motivated to succeed, your ANS can and will impose limitations on your performance. And because it operates autonomously, following hidden algorithms and protocols, your performance will always be somewhat unpredictable. Why do you do well in practice sessions but not in the game? Why do you have bad days? Why do conflict, weather, and what you ate for breakfast cause such wild fluctuations in what you accomplish? Because your autonomic nervous system has its own agenda and follows its own rules.

In the brain stem, where the top of the spinal cord intersects the brain, is a cone-shaped mass of neurons called the *medulla oblongata,* or simply the medulla for short. Above and just forward of that is an almond-sized part of the brain called the *hypothalamus*.

The medulla and hypothalamus serve as the command and control centers for the ANS. Anatomically, they are buried in the deep core of your brain, literally below the regions that govern conscious thought. Their anatomical position is also a metaphor because their operations lie beneath our conscious minds.

The medulla regulates a variety of functions for the ANS, including:

- Ventilation: the complex mechanical process of moving air into and out of the lungs.
- Respiration: the utilization of oxygen, balanced by removing carbon dioxide.
- Blood pressure and volume.
- Reflexes such as vomiting, coughing, sneezing, and swallowing.

The hypothalamus regulates the release of a variety of hormones (vasopressin, oxytocin, somatostatin, growth hormone-releasing hormone, etc.) that serve a wide range of functions, including:

- Thermoregulation (maintaining body temperature).
- Sexual differentiation, urges, and childbirth processes.
- Panting, sweating, and shivering.
- Blood pressure and heart rate.
- Gastrointestinal tract stimulation.
- Feeling hungry or full.
- Growth.
- Feelings: pleasure or happiness, fear, and stress.
- Circadian rhythms: waking up and falling to sleep.

As you can see, the command and control centers of the medulla and hypothalamus together regulate a complex range of functions and processes across the body and between its systems. But how are these brain regions connected to the rest of the body? How do they communicate, receive data, and send commands? Through a network of nerves.

Twelve cranial nerve bundles extend directly from the brain stem. The ANS has nerve fibers—think of them as trunk lines—through four of these. These direct connections control functions like pupil dilation and eye focusing (which we'll discuss in Chapter 10), tears, nasal mucus, saliva, and several organs in your chest and belly. In addition to these direct cranial nerve lines, the body has thirty-one spinal nerve bundles which are not connected directly to the brain but branch out from the spinal cord. They exit the spinal column at various points in your thorax (chest and upper back), lumbar region (lower back), and sacral region (tailbone). The ANS has nerve lines running through most of these bundles, which provide bi-directional communication between the command and control centers in the medulla and hypothalamus with organs in your thorax and abdomen. These nerve connections are composed of specialized cells: neurons, glial cells, nuclei, and ganglia. The ANS has dedicated nerve lines, so signals from the somatic or voluntary nerve system (SNS) won't get crossed with messages running through the ANS. Again, the ANS runs in the background or below the level of conscious thought.

Let's imagine some ways that the ANS can "mess with your game" (whatever that is) that aren't immediately obvious or directly observable to the untrained eye.

- Speeding up or slowing down pulse and respiration, affecting the volume and ratio of oxygen and carbon dioxide in your blood at any given moment, and thus how much power your brain and muscles have to perform.
- High blood pressure or low blood pressure.
- Reflexive responses to bright lights, loud noises, temperature changes, sudden movements, and perceived threats.

- Nervous energy, twitching, and fine motor skills.

- Depth perception and visually tracking objects.

- Isolating and discerning particular sounds, like speech, from background noise.

- Speeding up or slowing down how fast your nervous system sends and receives data between the parts of your body, affecting your precision and accuracy.

- Introducing extra data and distractions (noise) into your conscious and unconscious mind, robbing you of mental bandwidth and focus at critical moments.

- Managing (or mismanaging) the temperature control systems in your body, which could cause you to sweat too much, feel dehydrated, get thirsty, or get chills and shiver in your extremities.

- Under stress, you might have digestion issues, an upset stomach, feel like you need to urinate or defecate under stress, or become constipated.

- Flood your body with hormones, adrenaline, dopamine, or other chemicals that affect how well your body will perform tasks, especially under stress.

- Dramatic changes in mood or attitude or energy level, causing you to swing between excitement and depression, hyper-focus and distraction, fatigue and bursts of manic energy.

- Sexual arousal or lack thereof, and the ability to sexually perform or not.

That's only a partial list of how the ANS, running in the background, can affect your mind-body connection. As you read through that list, ask yourself how many of those would be, or have been, factors that affected your ability to perform your best and achieve your potential in work, sports, or the routine tasks of life. I suspect all of them have affected you at one time or another, at unpredictable times and in inconsistent ways. One day, you can't do anything wrong, but other days you feel like you can't do anything right. You don't know why. You criticize yourself. You question your body, your motivation, and your commitment. But the reality is that your body and mind can only work well together if they are synchronized. And if your ANS is not cooperating with your conscious mind and physical systems, your outcomes will be inconsistent and below your expectations.

In the next chapter, we'll discover the programming and protocols that the ANS uses to regulate your body and how those translate to better or worse performances.

CHAPTER 5
PRIME DIRECTIVE

If we can better coordinate the intricate dance between our conscious mind and unconscious body systems, we can perform more consistently and closer to our potential.

You probably have a smartphone. On it, you have "apps," programs that perform particular tasks, like mail, music, or maps. You probably have many running at the same time. In addition to those you chose to open, other apps are running in the background: searching for cell towers, location tracking, instant messaging apps, whatever. All these use up system resources like memory and battery. So, something has to tell them when to run and when to wait, allocating bandwidth and power between them. That system, underneath the apps, is the operating system. It follows priorities and protocols that drive your phone's performance and battery life.

The ANS is the deep operating system that synchronizes and directs the rest of your body's organs and systems. What are its priorities and protocols? How does it decide how to regulate everything from digestion to energy management and wound repair?

The ANS's prime directive is called homeostasis, derived from the Greek for "same state" or "same condition." Living things try to maintain a steady condition or return to their default settings. If you bend a plant over and then let go, it will try to return to an upright state, pointing at the sun. If you push my cat off her spot on the top of the sofa by the window, she'll climb back up. Living things try to regain homeostasis.

So the ANS works quietly in the background, trying to maintain homeostasis in your body. The ANS constantly receives data from around the body, updating it on conditions and alerting it to changes. It processes that data and decides what needs to happen in your body to maintain its default settings. Then it sends signals directing your organs and systems, coordinating their adjustments. If you break a bone or get infected, the other body systems work together to overcome or compensate for the injury. It's why you get a fever: the system detects invaders (bacteria) and raises the temperature to try and kill them off.

But sometimes, the ANS has to disrupt homeostasis in the short run to preserve it in the long run. In other words, it will initiate emergency procedures to keep you alive.

For example, suppose you fall out of your kayak into freezing water. You go under, and then your head pops above the surface. You gulp in a lung full of cold, wet air. You start losing heat rapidly through your damp skin and the humid air in your lungs.

The ANS, monitoring your body from millions of sensory points, becomes aware of the situation and determines that you're in crisis. The first thing it does is hit the emergency alarm button and send out a general alert. Think of a submarine movie, with the klaxons blaring, the red lights flashing, and the crew running to their battle stations. In your body, this is the "fight or flight" mode, and we'll talk about it a lot more in later chapters. But the ANS is the captain that sounds the alarm, letting the body's systems know that there is an emergency and to be ready to respond quickly.

Now that your body is on high alert, the ANS considers its options and consults its emergency procedures. The prime directive is homeostasis: maintain the body's default settings. But it's struggling because it can't generate enough heat throughout your body to keep every part at its ideal temperature. So, based on its deep programming, the ANS begins prioritizing. It decides that the highest priority is conserving energy for the core functions of your brain, heart, and lungs. It orders the blood vessels in your limbs and extremities to constrict, forcing warm, oxygenated blood back toward your core. It directs your heart to beat faster and your lungs to breathe more quickly, rapidly taking in as much oxygen and shedding as much CO_2 as possible.

It shuts down extraneous brain activity because the brain consumes an enormous amount of energy and calories, and the system doesn't have any to spare right now. It tells the brain to focus only on the immediate problem because this is not the time to compose poetry or think about your grocery list. It focuses your eyes and ears on the problem, so you get tunnel vision. All you can see is the water and the shore, and all you can think about is how to get out of this water as fast as possible. The digestive system locks down because it has no energy to spare, but it needs any ready sugars and electrolytes that you have in reserve. The ANS ignites the emergency generators in your muscle tissues, and cells start burning those resources to generate body heat. Back in your lungs, adjustments are made in the bronchial passages to filter the cold, wet air. Your glands are squirting adrenaline like the afterburners in a fighter jet, giving you the energy to stay at the surface and swim to shore.

We could go on, but you get the idea. The ANS monitors your body and its systems and follows the prime directive: *restore homeostasis immediately!* Failing that, it follows priority protocols and protects the critical organs, telling the rest to survive as best as possible until it can get around to them.

Now, this process is more noticeable when falling into freezing water. But the ANS is always working the same way. If you're secure, sleeping in your bed, the ANS monitors and maintains your systems to maintain homeostasis. If you're injured or stressed, it makes adjustments. If you are performing a task, whether mowing the lawn or quarterbacking the Super Bowl, the ANS is running in the background, regulating systems and resources, trying to keep the body in a healthy state.

And if maintaining homeostasis puts your ANS in conflict with what you think is most important, like passing your exam or beating your opponent, the ANS is going to win that battle every time because you don't have conscious control over it. It will initiate emergency procedures, divert energy, focus your senses and mental processes, recalibrate your pulse and respiration, and use a thousand other tricks to maintain what it believes to be your default state—even when you would gladly burn those resources to achieve your goal. Your conscious mind wants to close this deal, pass this test, win this race and would gladly suffer and sacrifice to do so. But your unconscious mind is running a different script. It doesn't care about bonuses, grades, and trophies, and it will regulate your systems to maintain core homeostasis, even if that means slowing down and inhibiting your performance. You will never perform consistently at your potential if your conscious mind conflicts with the priorities and programming of your ANS.

So, what can you do? Are you doomed to have inconsistent results forever? Well, yes and no.

On the one hand, the ANS exists for a reason: to keep you from seriously hurting yourself or even dying. Imagine running a 10k race, trying to beat your previous best time. It's hot and humid, and your body temperature is rising to dangerous levels. You might keep up the pace, ignoring all the warning signals from your body because your conscious mind wants to achieve its goal so badly. You might want it so badly that you fall over dead before the finish line. But your ANS has fail-safes built into it, so it starts making rapid adjustments, slowing you down for your own good. Your conscious will and unconscious ANS can run at cross purposes, and whenever they do, you won't perform your best.

But we can train our bodies to better collaborate with the ANS. We can't and shouldn't eliminate the fail-safes, but we can train them to respond more predictably and, to some degree, manage their responses. If we can better coordinate the intricate dance between our conscious mind and unconscious body systems, we can perform more consistently and closer to our potential.

But to do so, we need to take a closer look at the protocols it follows to keep you alive and operating.

CHAPTER 6
RESPONSE AND RESILIENCE

Dynamic resilience means adjusting the right amount at the correct times to help you consistently and safely perform at or near your potential in any given situation.

As we've seen, the nervous system is subdivided into the somatic (voluntary) and the autonomic (involuntary) systems, which have their command and control centers in the medulla and the hypothalamus. From those locations in the brain, the ANS operates via a complex network of dedicated nerve lines to the other organs and systems of the body.

But the ANS itself is made up of two equal, opposite, and complementary subsystems: the sympathetic and parasympathetic nervous systems. Understanding the division between these two halves of the ANS is the key to understanding how its programming and protocols affect performance.

The sympathetic system controls our reflexive actions, often called our fight or flight response: the high-speed, adrenaline-fueled reactions that take over in fires, car accidents, or being chased by wild animals. The parasympathetic system controls the body at rest: the even tempo that comes with recovery, digestion, and sleep.

The sympathetic and parasympathetic systems have dedicated anatomic components, like the accelerator and brake systems on your car. The accelerator pedal is connected to fuel lines, which run to the throttle on the engine. That system makes the car go fast. The brake pedals connect to brake lines, which run to the brakes on the wheels. That system slows the vehicle down. But they can also be thought of as modes of operation: go and slow.

The sympathetic system is your body's go mode. The accelerator pedal is in your brain stem, specific nerves are the fuel lines, and they run to particular organs or special tissues in those organs. When you shift into sympathetic mode, everything speeds up: thoughts, processes, and movements.

Why would you want to be in fight-or-flight mode? Because the ANS might determine that you need to fight or flee to preserve your life, health, and homeostasis. Consider your distant ancestor, leaving the comfort of his village to hunt for food. He's in a dangerous wilderness, surrounded by predators and enemies. His ANS shifts into sympathetic mode. He's hyper-alert, his brain cycling fast, dialed into his prey and any threats. His pulse and respiration speed up, ready to sprint toward or away from danger. His metabolism is racing, ready to deliver energy to his muscles. He's sweating to maintain his body temperature through his exertions. When his prey is in sight, or an enemy attacks him, he reacts instantly, either leaping forward for the kill or running away to safety.

Suppose your ancestor successfully takes his prey and drags the elk back to his village. As the village welcomes him, his body shifts into parasympathetic mode. His heart and lungs slow back down, and he stops sweating. His mind and his muscles relax. They prepare the game and enjoy a feast. After eating his fill, he lies back in his bed. The ANS obeys its prime directive to maintain life, health, and homeostasis by digesting his dinner, replenishing his energy reserves, and healing any injuries. For these reasons, the parasympathetic mode is sometimes called the rest and digest response.

Your ANS constantly works the accelerator and the brakes, switching between go and slow modes. They aren't good or bad. Both are equally necessary, depending on the situation. Your ANS constantly monitors your environment and status and adjusts the body's organs and systems accordingly. It takes in data through your five sensory systems (touch, taste, sight, sound, and smell) like the flight computer of an advanced aircraft monitors the plane's sensor arrays. And just as the flight computer adjusts the aircraft's systems based on preprogrammed protocols, your ANS shifts between the go and slow modes through its sympathetic and parasympathetic subsystems. If the airplane faces a headwind, it might subtly adjust fuel consumption rates in the engines to compensate for the longer flying time. If your ANS perceives you are in danger, it will enact emergency procedures by sending signals to your organs to compensate. It's always trying to keep the body in homeostasis, to protect and preserve your life.

So if it's hot outside, the ANS tells the pores to open up, sweat to cool the skin, and capillaries to move blood closer to the skin, shedding internal heat to maintain body temperature at 98.6 F. The ANS reads the environmental cues of the daylight/dark cycle and tells the glands when to release melatonin to make us sleepy so that our brains and organs can rest. The ANS reacts to danger by flooding our system with adrenaline so we can fight or flee to safety. Imagine you're sleeping peacefully when the smoke alarm goes off in your house in the middle of the night. You're instantly alert, although you might be groggy as you try to figure out what's happening. But it doesn't take long: within moments, you grasp what the alarm means and smell smoke. Now adrenaline is pumping through your body, and sleep is the furthest thing from your mind. You're hyper-focused and run to your children's bedrooms, making rapid decisions at twice your normal speed. That's what the ANS can do when it kicks into fight or flight mode; at times, our survival depends on that ability.

Sometimes, it can become overwhelmed by confusing environmental stimuli or emotional stresses, including unpredictable changes or chaotic circumstances. Sudden loud noises and bright lights will kick it into sympathetic mode, even if there's no real danger. Imagine a football player in a crowded stadium. The stadium lights, flashing scoreboards, and the crowd shouting as loud as a jet engine can overwhelm the ANS and put the player into fight or flight mode, even if he's trying to calm himself down to kick a field goal.

Sometimes, chemical imbalances caused by diet, hormonal imbalances, drugs, and alcohol can shift the body into either sympathetic or parasympathetic mode at inappropriate times. Imagine someone under the influence of alcohol or marijuana behind the wheel of a car. They ought to be alert, but they've shifted into slow mode. Their thought processes and reflexes are dangerously mismatched to their actual situation.

We can keep imagining scenarios when your ANS might put you in the wrong mode at the wrong time. The student taking a test gets stressed and goes into fight or flight mode when she needs to slow down and focus. After lunch, you sit in a work meeting, and your mind wanders when you should be taking notes. You make a bad shot on the golf course and get angry with yourself instead of letting it go and resetting your system for the next shot. You argue with your spouse and then can't focus on your child's needs. The pilot loses an engine and panics instead of working on the problem. The nurse runs too fast all shift and misreads the instructions on the patient's chart.

Each of these events causes a cascade of effects throughout your organs and systems as the ANS blasts signals and pumps hormones, trying to keep up with changing demands. And most of the inconsistencies in your performance, whether at work or on the playing field, come from your body being unconsciously out of sync with your conscious goals. These mismatches result in mental lapses, missed instructions, vision problems, upset stomachs, sweating and shakes and tics, impaired motor control, exhaustion, and needing to pee at the worst possible moments.

So, what can you do about it? How can you gain greater control over when and how your ANS shifts gears? That's what the rest of this book is about, but I must caution you: you will never gain total control. Nor should you, because the ANS's complex systems and protocols are there to keep you alive and healthy. Without them, you might forget to breathe, digest, or adjust your body temperature.

But you can train your ANS to respond more appropriately and consistently to environmental and psychological demands. You can indirectly influence it by recognizing when it is switching modes and interrupting that process. And you can strengthen your body's systems so that they are less likely to trigger autonomous protocols.

The goal is to make your ANS and its responses more resilient to stress and change. I call that "dynamic resilience" because you don't want your ANS stuck in any constant state. That would be like having non-responsive accelerator or brake pedals in your car, which could get you killed. You want a highly responsive ANS, but not one over or under-reacting. Think about driving down a twisting road: if your car is over-steering or under-steering, swerving too much or too little to match the turns, you're going to hit a tree or go off a cliff. You want to make appropriate turns, hitting the gas or the break just enough to turn smoothly and accurately.

We all live with rapid, constant change in our environment and the demands placed on us. Dynamic resilience means adjusting the right amount at the correct times to help you consistently and safely perform at or near your potential in any given situation.

So, how can we harden our conscious and unconscious brain-body connections to become dynamically resilient? To do so, we need more than estimates and feelings about how we're doing. We need measurable data about what is happening inside our bodies and brains.

CHAPTER 7
MEASURING THE MIND

The ANS is hardwired into you, so you can't turn it off. However, we can teach it to be more responsive and resilient and, in some ways, to override its programming, like switching your transmission into manual mode.

What is "normal" behavior? How do you know if you are consistently performing near your potential?

Consider evaluating "physical fitness." Suppose we randomly select people off the street and rate each person as either "fit" or "fat." But how do we define our terms—what is "fit" and what is "fat?" Those are relative ideas: fit compared to whom? An Olympic athlete? Their next-door neighbor? People from hundreds of years ago? The center of the bell curve in our sample?

Suppose we define fitness as having a resting pulse of fewer than 60 beats per minute (bpm) with no more than 25% body fat. If we tested 50 random strangers, measuring and recording their pulse and body fat percentages, we'd quickly discover a great deal of variability between individuals. Some will have pulses as low as 48 bpm and some as high as 90 bpm. Each person's numbers may vary significantly from one day to the next or even between different times of the day. We'd also be surprised that surface appearances are only marginally predictive of these measurements. A big, hulking football player might have a lower body fat percentage and resting pulse than an average-sized woman, and a thin man might have a strained heart. You can only sometimes tell a book by its cover. We have to open it and read what's inside.

Because the brain is so complex, behaviors and inconsistent performances can have various causes. In much of medicine, measurement is quantitative: blood tests provide objective numbers which physicians can compare with established norms. Establishing a baseline for "normal" or your "potential normal" would require us to measure something capable of being quantified. We can count how many times your heart beats in a minute, how fast you can run a mile, or how many math problems you can complete in a minute. But how do we measure factors that affect performance, like "focus" or "execution?"

Until the last few decades, we had no practical, effective way to measure brain activity. Renaissance anatomists like Leonardo DaVinci dissected cadavers and produced detailed drawings of anatomical structures. Every college student who has studied anatomy and physiology is familiar with the famous textbook Gray's Anatomy. Published in 1858, it proves that even in the mid-nineteenth century, we knew a fantastic amount about the structures of the body and its organs. We even learned a lot about the brain's anatomy: its two hemispheres, folds and ridges, and the nerve bundles leading in and out.

While the heart is a mechanical pump triggered and regulated by electrical signals, the brain has no moving parts. Like a giant circuit board made up of microprocessors, it functions purely through electricity. Therefore, to understand how the brain is working at any given moment, we have to measure the electrical signals traveling through it. And because it's tucked safely in your skull, until recently, we had no technology that allowed us to watch a live brain in action.

But our tools for measuring and diagnosing the brain are getting better. In the 21st century, we're entering a golden age of data collection. New tools allow us to measure body functions that weren't observable with prior technology. And this lets us see connections between organs, systems, and symptoms. We're learning that the body is far more integrated than we ever realized, that disease is more systemic, and that we must consider the possibility of unintended consequences when treating illness.

In the early 1990s, I was involved with numerous clinical studies, integrating neuropsychological testing with treating diseases that our compartmentalized medical system would never suspect had a neurological connection. I did a lot of work, in more than a dozen clinics, with cystic fibrosis, sickle cell anemia, and post-cancer patients. We would see them annually after their initial diagnosis and treatment and assess neuropsychological functioning.

We have better tools now, but in a decade or two, we'll look at them the same way we do black-and-white sonograms from the 1980s. As testing technologies improve, we'll discover more complex and quantifiable relationships between the brain and the body, especially those connections hidden within the autonomic nervous system.

Medical technology has advanced to scientifically and objectively measure brain and nervous system performance. We don't need to rely on subjective descriptions by patients or those around them because we can look at brain metrics using *electroencephalogram* (EEG) technology. Just as an electrocardiogram (EKG/ECG) measures electrical pulses through the heart and allows us to diagnose cardiac irregularities, an EEG measures the electrical signals through various brain regions, revealing patterns and changes.

All electromagnetic waves, including brain waves, have frequencies, and frequencies are measured in units called hertz (Hz). Imagine a wave pattern, a series of peaks and valleys, flowing from left to right on a screen in front of you. Draw a vertical line down the screen through one of the peaks and run a stopwatch for precisely one second. The number of peaks that pass by your line during that second is the frequency of that wave. If twenty cycles of the wave go past in one second, that's a 20 Hz wave.

Now, imagine the shape of that 20 Hz wave compared to that of a 100 Hz wave. For more peaks and valleys to go past your line in one second, the slopes between the peaks and valleys will be steeper. The higher the frequency, the more jagged and cramped the waves appear. A lower frequency will appear more gently rounded, almost lazily looping along.

Brain waves are given names based on their frequency: Alpha, Beta, Gamma, and so on. Delta waves are the lowest frequencies, less than 4 Hz (very slow, with a long slope between the peaks and valleys). They are dominant in newborn infants and adults in a deep sleep. Delta waves indicate that the brain is detached or resting from monitoring the outside world. Theta Waves have a frequency of between 4 and 8 Hz, indicating that the brain is running slow, even half asleep, daydreaming, pondering, or creating. Faster frequencies between 8 and 12 Hz are known as Alpha waves, associated with imagination and creativity. When the brain starts accelerating, it produces Beta waves. We differentiate between Low Beta, between 12-20 Hz, and High Beta at 20 Hz and above. As the brain gets closer to High Beta, it moves into sympathetic, or fight-or-flight, mode. It's intensely focused on the perceived emergency and trying to solve the life-and-death problem it believes that it is facing (even if our conscious mind has exaggerated or imagined the problem). It's akin to what's going on in Obsessive Compulsive Disorder (OCD). The brain has become hyper-aware of the environment. It processes input rapidly and quickly adjusts the body's organs and systems. This is okay if it's appropriate for the situation, such as a crisis or conflict requiring quick and decisive action (a bear attack or burning building). Finally, Gamma waves are the fastest, in frequencies above 30 hertz. These represent highly integrated concentration, information-rich processing, and intense memory recall or problem-solving. A brain taking a challenging exam might have some Gamma waves running through it as it tries to recall the study material and solve the problems or answer the questions under timed conditions.

To be clear, the brain never has only one frequency of wave running through it at a time. Multiple wave patterns move through complex neural pathways in different locations, controlling various functions. But at any given moment, one frequency will be dominant at a given area: so, you might have more High Beta and less Theta running through the left hemisphere of your brain, while in the right hemisphere, there is more Low Beta. The EEG connections (or "leads") on the skull measure the ratios between these waves and determine which frequencies are dominant at a particular time and place.

These waves are like the gears in your car: you need them all, but the challenge is to be in the right gear at the right time. If you're going up a hill, you don't want to be stuck in high gear, or you won't have enough low-end torque to climb. And you can't cruise down the interstate at 70 mph in first gear, or your engine will explode. You can decide when to shift gears if you have a manual transmission (a stick shift). But most of us have automatic transmissions, which means that a computer decides when to shift gears. And that's an excellent way to think of brainwaves, focus, and the mind-body connection because the ANS is like your automatic transmission. But if it's putting your brain into the wrong gear, you're out of rhythm for the situation.

For example, if you're trying to sink a putt to win your golf match, you want to run some Alpha waves of 10-12 Hz or some Low Betas for concentration without triggering sympathetic mode. But if the stress of the putt has accelerated you closer to 20 Hz and High Beta, then your ANS has shifted into sympathetic. You become over-focused, even obsessive, over the putt. Your perception becomes tunnel-visioned, your thinking becomes more black-and-white and less creative, and your fine-muscle coordination decreases as adrenaline floods your large muscles. In short, it becomes more difficult to judge and execute the right line and speed for the putt. You misread, pull, and run it past the hole.

On the flip side, if you're driving a twisty mountain road at night in a snowstorm, you need to be as alert as possible with your reflexes ready to react. It's probably a bad time for your ANS to have shifted into a completely parasympathetic, "rest and digest" mode, with many low-frequency Theta waves lulling you into complacency, daydreaming, and maybe even sleepiness. What you want in this situation is Low Beta: the alertness that comes in the 12-20 Hz range, staying just below the threshold where fight-or-flight kicks in because you can't sustain that level of controlled panic for the hour or two it takes to get to the ski resort.

If your body were a car with a stick shift, your conscious mind would select the right gear for your situation and goals. The ANS is hardwired into you, so you can't turn it off. However, we can teach it to be more responsive and resilient and, in some ways, to override its programming, like switching your transmission into manual mode.

CHAPTER 8
FREQUENCY AND FOCUS

If a balanced and composed ANS and increased SMR waves can help a cat catch a mouse, an NFL quarterback throw a pass, or a fighter pilot execute complex maneuvers at over five hundred miles per hour, doesn't it stand to reason that they can help you to perform more consistently near your potential?

What do Cats and Quarterbacks have in common? Uncommon focus.

Have you ever watched a cat stare at a spot where it knows a mouse is hiding, perhaps behind a cabinet or under a piece of furniture? The cat's tail twitches slightly, but the rest of its body is at ease as it gazes intently. This might go on for twenty minutes. The cat seems almost asleep. But the moment the mouse appears, the cat moves like lightning. Its relaxed muscles release coiled energy with quick and deadly accuracy. How could it sit still for so long, alert and focused?

An NFL quarterback has three seconds to do his job. As soon as the ball is snapped, twenty-two big men begin moving very quickly. The quarterback takes a few steps back. He hears grunts and groans, bodies smashing, and a hundred thousand fans screaming as loudly as a jet engine. Opponents are rushing into his peripheral vision, threatening a sack, a fumble, or a concussion—maybe all three. Despite all this, he has to focus downfield, tracking his receivers and their defenders. He has to calculate their angles and speeds, anticipating their movements. Sorting through this maelstrom of noise and data, he must make the right decision and act immediately. The average time from snap to release in the NFL is 2.8 seconds. His brain must scan, digest, and process while his body moves, reacts, and acts—all in less time than it takes you to say, "One Mississippi, Two Mississippi, Three Mississippi." How does he do it?

When it comes time to perform some task, your conscious mind says, *Pay attention! Stay focused on this exam, this project, this putt!* If your mind-body connection is strong, if you have strengthened and trained your brain to coordinate with your ANS, you will maintain focus, and your heart, lungs, and other organs will drop into an optimal zone.

But if that connection is weak, your attention will wander. You'll be distracted by street noises outside the window, by people talking around you, by the last putt that you missed, by the scoreboard, by the noise of the stadium crowd waving towels and doing "the wave."

What makes that connection stronger or weaker? As we saw in the last chapter, focus is a function of brainwaves. With no moving parts, the brain operates by electromagnetic waves racing through its hundred billion neurons and trillions of synapses at hundreds of miles per hour across very short distances.

So why do cats and quarterbacks have an uncommon capacity to focus? Because they have well-regulated autonomic nervous systems. Their sympathetic and parasympathetic systems are balanced, working in harmony. Why? The answer lies in a story about cats, the space race, and secret rocket fuels.

In 1968, Dr. Barry Sterman, a neuroscientist at the University of California Los Angeles (UCLA), was experimenting with cat brains. He hooked the cats up to an EEG monitor. Sterman discovered that when the cats' brains hit a very particular frequency, somewhere around 12-15 Hz, the wave took on an unusual shape. The top of the wave would sort of flatten out for a few seconds, like a plateau. It would seem to drift in this elevated state, like a golf ball that catches the wind at the top of its trajectory and gets carried for an extra twenty yards of distance. On his EEG printouts (in 1968, the monitors printed out long strips of paper), these 12-15 Hz waves were very distinct and intriguing. They weren't Alpha, Beta, or any other known wave. Sterman called this wave pattern sensory motor rhythm, or SMR.

Dr. Sterman wondered whether he could encourage these waves, and he discovered that he could. He reinforced the pattern with rewards using operant conditioning techniques while the cats were connected to the EEG monitor. Like Pavlov's dogs, after a while, the cats' brains not only produced SMR waves on demand, they dropped quickly into them as a sort of default state.

A short time later, Sterman got a research grant from NASA. It was the height of the space race, and the government was worried that rocket fuel fumes could cause seizures in astronauts and ground crews. To save money, Sterman decided to use the cats he already had in his lab. He exposed them to the dangerous chemical fuel hydrazine and recorded the results. About half the cats had predictable seizures. But the rest seemed almost immune. Sterman couldn't figure out why. What was different about these cats that protected their systems from seizures? They began looking more closely at these special cats. They even dissected some of them to discover whether there might be some physiological explanation. But he and his research assistants didn't find any significant difference between the cats that seized and those that didn't. They looked at the individual cats' histories. Where did they come from? When had they arrived at the UCLA labs? Had they been exposed to some environmental influence in a special section of the lab? Had they had the same diet? What previous experiments had they been exposed to?

Then it occurred to someone in the lab that the cats nearly immune to the seizures had been the same ones used in the sensory motor rhythm experiments. The cats that reacted severely to the hydrazine hadn't been a part of that test group. Somehow, the cats whose brains had been trained to develop SMR patterns had developed more resilient nervous systems, more resistant to seizures, than those that hadn't. It was the only difference that they could discover.

Sterman realized that he was on to something. After additional research, he used EEG monitoring to train one of his lab assistants to develop consistent SMR wave patterns. This woman had a history of uncontrolled seizures and thus had never been able to obtain a driver's license. The results were dramatic. His lab assistant's seizures declined so much that she was able to get a California driver's license.

With this, the field of EEG feedback was launched. We can measure brain activity and train the brain to become stronger, like we train the cardiovascular or skeletal-muscular systems. We can develop stronger brains, not by behavior modification or "talking therapy" but by teaching the brain to operate in optimal wave patterns.

How can the NFL quarterback on the run read all the complex variables of time, speed, and distance, analyze them in real-time, make a decision, and then execute it with a well-thrown pass in less time than it takes you to read this sentence? How does a classical pianist or jazz guitarist close their eyes and play for thirty minutes without sheet music, improvising, adapting, and harmonizing with other musicians in real-time? How does a dogfighting fighter pilot, with g-forces pulling at her bones and pushing the blood out of her brain, keep track of the ground, other planes and missiles, and the array of instruments in her cockpit? They have all developed SMR brainwave patterns that help them function in "The Zone."

Of course, there is an alternative, but it's not very good. The quarterback, musician, or fighter pilot could accelerate the brain above 20 Hz into the High Beta zone. They could do that with stimulants like caffeine or even amphetamines like Adderall. That would trigger the hyper-focused controlled panic of the sympathetic state when a dump truck swerves over the center line or when a big dog starts chasing you on your morning run. But that comes with a pretty high cost, as you know if you ever had a dump truck barreling down on you or a dog snapping at your heels. At that moment, there are no Alpha waves in your brain, meaning you have zero creativity or imagination and are just reacting. Your adrenal glands spray adrenaline and cortisol into your bloodstream, providing the hyper focus and lightning-fast reflexes you need to swerve or sprint. But that rocket fuel has a very short burn. Within a few minutes, your energy level will crash and crash hard. Have you ever narrowly avoided a car crash? How did you feel 5 minutes later? Were your hands shaking? Was your heart still racing? Did you feel completely exhausted? Did it take you hours, if not days, to fully recover? Sometimes it's necessary to pull the brain's fire alarm. But it's a terrible strategy for managing responsibilities or challenges for more than a few minutes.

The quarterbacks or fighter pilots of the past might not have had formal EEG feedback training. However, it is becoming more and more common in professional sports, the military, and executive suites. Until now, people naturally gifted with higher SMR levels probably reinforced them informally: they learned what "The Zone" felt like and taught themselves to get into it through breathing, meditation, and other concentration techniques. Darwinian natural selection allowed those with naturally strong SMR waves to outperform rivals and rise to the top of their professions.

Today, we can measure and calculate the ratios between these various waves and know at what ranges the brain performs best. These ranges aren't subjective guesses any more than saying that your blood pressure should be below 120/80 or that your ideal cholesterol ratio ought to be about 3.5:1. Respiration is also critical because it oxygenates the brain. If we breathe too slowly, our brain doesn't get enough fuel, and we fall asleep. Fast, shallow breathing prevents the respiratory and circulatory systems from synchronizing and properly oxygenating the brain. Ideally, we want to take 6-8 deep breaths, from the diaphragm, per minute at rest.

For the brain, the EEG ratios that will provide the strongest brain-body connection for consistent performance are:

- High Beta = < 1.4 (High Beta:SMR) at rest.
- Theta = 2.0 - 2.7 (Theta:Low Beta) at rest.

Those crazy, lazy plateaus in SMR waves increase creativity and processing speed. They kept seizures at bay in cats and an epileptic lab assistant because when the brain is in its sweet spot, the ANS is more robust and better able to resist tension and disease. A strong body begins with a strong brain.

But here's the question you must ask yourself: if a balanced and composed ANS and increased SMR waves can help a cat catch a mouse, an NFL quarterback throw a pass, or a fighter pilot execute complex maneuvers at over five hundred miles per hour, doesn't it stand to reason that they can help you to perform more consistently near your potential?

CHAPTER 9
COHERENT POWER

Whether you're competing in an athletic event, teaching school, or racing through the airport to catch your plane, you don't want to be out of breath, exhausted, with your brain racing from stress. Conditioning your system to engage resonant breathing that triggers coherent power will help you be the best version of yourself.

How do you move? It's not a simple question with a simple answer. Animal movement is incredible, and human movement is even more so. For a long time, scientists and engineers worked to develop computers that could beat a human grandmaster at chess, and they did it. But, as of yet, no one has taught a robot to move and to keep learning to move in real-time like an 8-year-old human.

Because whether it's small movements like blinking your eyes or turning the page or large movements like running, jumping, or lifting, your muscle tissues function through a complex series of chemical reactions inside individual muscle cells. One of the most important is the Citric Acid Cycle (or Krebs Cycle). Carbohydrates, fats, and proteins stored inside the cell are converted to energy, catalyzed by oxygen through either aerobic or anaerobic respiration. Your muscle cells get the oxygen they need to generate power and motion because it is exchanged for carbon dioxide in the alveoli sacs in your lungs and transported on red blood cells, which travel through your circulatory system like tiny delivery trucks.

So, every move you make depends upon a complex dance involving your cardiovascular, respiratory, and muscular systems, delivering power where and when you need it. All of the dancers must be tightly synchronized to provide maximum, reliable power on demand.

Missteps between the dancers can rob you of power. If your heart is beating out of synch with your lungs, the critical exchange of oxygen for carbon dioxide will be less efficient. If your blood pressure rises too high or falls too low, a hardwired loop in your autonomic nervous system called the baroreflex slows down or speeds up your heart to maintain homeostasis. Your ANS also regulates blood pressure changes by commanding your heart and kidneys to release certain hormones into the bloodstream. It will speed up or slow down your brain waves or fire them through different neural pathways. Depending on whether your ANS has shifted into sympathetic or parasympathetic mode, it will use all the tools in its toolbox to obey its prime directive and maintain homeostasis. In the ANS's programming, homeostasis takes higher priority than providing your muscles with maximum power on demand. Providing the extra energy to sprint the last mile of your 10k or to lift another set are secondary or tertiary considerations. Your conscious mind wants to achieve your goals, but your unconscious ANS stays focused on keeping you alive by adjusting systems to maintain blood pressure, body temperature, etc. And that's why your muscles sometimes run out of gas at the worst possible moments.

Long-term stress—from psychological pressure, environmental factors, or disease—can degrade the ability of your systems to respond appropriately and quickly. You can get stuck in one gear: high blood pressure, weak muscles, and poor concentration. You can't adjust to meet the demands of the situation.

There will always be somebody stronger, faster, and with more endurance than you. Your challenge is to consistently deliver as much power to your muscles as you are capable of generating.

You can train your body systems to stay synchronized, even under physical or psychological stress. I call that coherent power, and you can develop it so that it's available on demand. To do so, we can use a technique called resonant frequency breathing.

We discussed how waves are measured in frequencies in the last chapter. Everything is subtly vibrating, or oscillating, at some frequency because its various molecules have natural motion. This is called the natural frequency of a system. Whenever force is applied to the system (wind blowing against it, water flowing over it, or electrical signals running through it), that introduces another frequency. If the natural frequency and the applied frequency match, they become resonant. The waves' amplitude (the height difference between the peaks and valleys) increases dramatically. Resonance is the sweet spot when a system is functioning most efficiently.

The cardiovascular and respiratory systems have natural frequencies coded into them. This coding triggers the ANS to initiate its programmed protocols, like the baroreflex we mentioned above. But if we can match our breathing and heart rates to the system's natural frequencies, they achieve resonant frequency and become much more efficient than usual. Thus resonance, or coherence, keeps our ANS from shifting gears and delivers maximum, reliable power to our muscles. And this triggers lower-frequency brain waves, dropping from Beta to Alpha, or even Theta. We feel strong, calm, and in control. And that allows us to perform at or near our potential consistently.

The good news is that we can use technology to find your resonant frequency and operant conditioning to teach your body to maintain it. We can't directly change the programming of our ANS, but we can indirectly influence it by avoiding its triggers and bypassing its emergency protocols. When we train our heart, lungs, and brain to be better coordinated, our body hums along in sync, and we can deliver coherent, focused, and consistent power to our muscles.

Now, this isn't magic. It doesn't allow us to exceed our muscular potential. It won't let you do pull-ups like a Navy SEAL unless you've developed that capacity. But it will let you do as many pull-ups as your muscles can without your body panicking, running out of gas, and shutting down.

How do we hack the ANS into increasing our capacity for coherent power? We begin with our breathing because that's the closest thing we have to a dial that we can turn, at will, with conscious effort. Most of us can't just choose to slow down our hearts with the power of our minds. To the extent that we can lower our pulse on demand, we do it by breathing deeper and slower, which triggers a cardiac response. When stressed, we breathe shallowly from the muscles around our rib cage. Because shallow breaths trade less oxygen for carbon dioxide in each breath, we have to take more breaths per minute to keep the CO_2 from building up in our system. The heart has to beat faster to keep up, moving the gasses into and out of our bloodstream. This response loop has a dynamic relationship with our ANS. Rapid, shallow breathing can trigger the sympathetic system protocols. So, we can put ourselves into panic mode by not taking in enough oxygen. But these responses can also be initiated by the ANS shifting into fight or flight mode: your brain waves speed up, and so does your breathing.

But diaphragmatic breathing initiates the opposite feedback loop. The diaphragm consists of the internal muscles between our thorax and abdomen (above the stomach and below the lungs). Inhaling and exhaling using these muscles fills and empties our lungs more completely, increasing the amount of oxygen exchanged for carbon dioxide. More air moved in each breath means that we need to take fewer breaths per minute. Again, this is dynamically responsive to our parasympathetic system: brain waves, respiration, and pulse all slow down.

Natural respiration frequency varies between individuals depending on age, fitness, etc., but generally, it lies somewhere between 4.5 and 6 breaths per minute. So when we breathe deeply from our diaphragm, taking about 10-12 seconds to inhale-exhale, our respiration frequency begins to harmonize with our body's natural frequency, bringing about resonance. And with resonance, our respiration becomes much more efficient.

In turn, our heart begins to slow down to match it. One measure of cardiac health is heart rate variability (HRV). When we take our pulse, we measure how many times our heart beats in a minute, but HRV measures how quickly it can adjust to changing demands. We want our hearts to accelerate or decelerate smoothly to meet our body's demands. If you're running up stairs, it needs to beat faster to move oxygen to your muscles more rapidly, but you don't want it pumping that fast when you're sleeping. When you carry groceries into the house, your heart should be able to pick up its pace just enough to send extra red blood cells to your leg muscles, then slow down when you finish.

And you want your respiration and pulse to sync with your brain wave frequencies. They should be able to march together in rhythm. This synchronization is known as coherence, and it produces coherent power.

Suppose I connect you to devices that monitor your respiration, pulse, and brainwaves and observe those measurements for 3 minutes. I want to see how long you can maintain resonant breathing and coherence between your lungs, heart, and brain. If you can only keep coherence for 30 seconds out of the 3 minutes, your muscles aren't going to have the consistent power on demand that you need to perform at or near your potential. But if you can train your system to manage these feedback loops at will and stay coherent for 2.5 of the 3 minutes, you'll notice dramatic improvements in your available power. Whether you're competing in an athletic event, teaching school, or racing through the airport to catch your plane, you don't want to be out of breath, exhausted, with your brain racing from stress. Conditioning your system to engage resonant breathing that triggers coherent power will help you be the best version of yourself.

CHAPTER 10
PRECISE COORDINATION

Converging and diverging our eyes, processing that information, and then acting on it is a complex task that requires precise coordination of a chain of muscles, organs, nervous systems, and processes within the body. The good news is that, with training and technology, we can strengthen those muscles and organs and teach ourselves to process inputs faster and more accurately.

Most submarines don't have windows. Instead, they have arrays of various kinds of sensors. If those sensors stop working or stop being reliable, the sub will blunder about dangerously in the dark ocean. You also have sensor arrays: vision, hearing, touch, taste, and smell. If they degrade or are no longer well-calibrated with your conscious mind, your performance at almost every task in life will suffer. People can lose one of their senses and still perform admirably (there are some remarkable blind and deaf athletes). But there's a crucial difference between losing a sense like vision and having it be simply unreliable. The blind person develops her other senses and leans on them to take up the slack. But the person who doesn't know that her vision is poorly-calibrated will find school and sports difficult without ever really understanding why. Others might label them as learning disabled or not athletic without realizing what's actually going on.

The quality of your mind-body connection is directly proportional to the quality of the data that your mind receives about the outside world through its sensory systems.

It's hard to read a book if the words look fuzzy or your eyes hurt after just a few minutes. Double vision makes it tough to pick your keys up off the floor or drive between the lane lines. Police officers struggle to quickly and accurately assess situations full of rapid movements between bright lights and shadows. And it's almost impossible to hit or catch a fast-moving ball if your eye can't track its motion in real-time.

When your senses are not well-calibrated, your brain will have to work harder to figure out what's going on, inform your conscious mind, and then relay your decisions back to the various parts of your body to respond in time to react. You'll struggle to read or study, make tragic mistakes during emergencies, and strike out at the plate more often. The consequences won't only be poor grades, car accidents, or lost games, but also headaches, confusion, and stress—not to mention stress-related illnesses and other consequences.

Imagine you're holding the latest, most fantastic smartphone camera. When you take a photo, there are two phases of decision-making involved. Phase I is conscious: you choose your subject, point the camera in that direction, and push the button. But Phase II is autonomous, outside your conscious control. Because as soon as you pointed the camera in the intended direction, its sensors began registering the amount of light and shadows, and its focusing mechanisms (nowadays either laser, LiDAR, or both) detected the distance to the target. When you consciously pushed the button, the software in its microprocessor chips made calculations at nearly the speed of light, adjusting hardware (including determining whether or how much of the flashlight to activate) and the exposure time. All of that was recorded, with more image processing, and the photo was stored in the camera's brain.

In the same way, there are conscious and unconscious phases to your vision. You consciously choose where to look, but you don't consciously operate the mechanisms of your eyes. Light is focused through the cornea without conscious thought or decision-making. It moves through an adjustable aperture known as the iris, which opens or closes to admit more or less light. It then passes through a lens into a cavity filled with a jellylike substance known as vitreous humor before hitting specialized photoreceptor cells in the retina, known as rods and cones. All these structures are fed by oxygen arriving through blood vessels, instantly and intricately adjusted by electrical signals and various amino acids known as peptides. All of this happens without you thinking about it. You look, they act, and you see.

But our analogy breaks down at this point because your phone only stores the image. On the other hand, you have to digest that information, make decisions, and then command your body to carry them out. Once the light hits the photoreceptors in your retina, that information is routed through nerves to various parts of your brain. This routing is complex and involves preprogrammed protocols. Specific images are classified as priority data (*A ball is about to hit your head! A deer just jumped in front of your car!*) and routed to unconscious decision centers, which initiate unconscious emergency reflexes (*Duck! Swerve!*). Other images are processed just as quickly but routed to conscious decision-making centers (*That pitch is low and outside, the count is three balls and one strike, so let's not swing at this one*).

All of this has to happen very quickly. In the case of baseball, a fastball takes 0.4 seconds to travel from the pitcher's hand to home plate. But it takes 0.1 seconds for the image of the moving ball to travel through the batter's eye and up the nerves to his brain. It takes another 0.15 seconds for the decision to be relayed down from his brain to his muscles. If you do the math, that leaves only 0.15 seconds for the batter's brain to analyze the pitch and make a decision.

Everything that we've talked about in this book up to now comes into play here. The autonomic nervous system operates the components of the eye. The ANS's sympathetic and parasympathetic systems regulate processing speed, reflexes, and how the other organs and systems in the body respond. Consistent performance at or near our potential is a function of our conscious will's mastery of our unconscious body. While it's easy to see how this dramatically affects our ability to hit fastballs or dodge deer on the highway, it impacts almost everything else we do.

To understand why, consider that we don't have just one eye, like a camera with one lens. Humans, and almost all animals, have binocular stereopsis. Because we have two eyes, we see in stereo, which is why we can perceive depth, the relative distance between objects nearer or further from us.

Stereoscopic vision requires the structures of the eye to make precise adjustments and the brain to do some tricky processing. Your right eye sends an image to the brain, and the left sends a slightly different image because it sees the world from 2.5 inches to the side. Without ocular mechanical adjustments and neural processing, the brain would register two distinct images, slightly misaligned. That's why, when you drink too much alcohol and your electrical-mechanical processes slow down and get sloppy, you get double vision so that your friend at the bar appears to have two heads.

For this discussion, let's look at two of the adjustments our visual systems have to make for us to see in stereo: convergence and divergence.

Hold your thumb out at arm's length and adjust your eyes so that it's in focus. Now relax your eye muscles so that it gradually falls out of focus. Do you see two thumbs? If so, then the images from your two eyes are not aligned accurately to form one image. Now, bring your thumb back into focus and slowly move it closer to the bridge of your nose. You may have to make some effort to keep it in focus so that it still looks like only one thumb because your two eyes need to smoothly converge their focal points to maintain the stereo image of a moving object. At some point, as your thumb nears the bridge of your nose, you'll lose focus and the stereo image because as your thumb gets into the gap between the eyes, and they can no longer converge enough to maintain it.

Convergence requires the autonomic nervous system, which controls many of the unconscious mechanisms of the eye, to work with the visual processing centers of the brain. How precisely and quickly they converge will determine how well you can see and how hard you have to work to see well, especially moving objects or in a rapidly changing environment. If you're studying books and papers, working at a computer screen, or making something with your hands, your eyes constantly have to converge. And when your system has to work too hard to converge, it makes mistakes and produces stress and exhaustion. It can shift your brain and organs into sympathetic panic mode. Your heart and lungs react, you begin sweating, and your task becomes much more demanding. You have to stop more often, and you get headaches.

To see things further away, especially objects moving away from you, requires the eyes to diverge. Hold something like a ball in one hand close to your face, and focus on it. Your eyes have converged, and your brain has merged the two images. Now, toss it across the room while trying to keep it in focus as it flies. To do that, your eyes had to shift from converging on the near object to mechanically diverging, processing the two rapidly changing images while keeping them aligned.

You do this all day long, looking down at your phone, then back up again. Drivers glance down at the fuel gauge or the GPS, then back up at the road. A student looks up at the teacher or the whiteboard and back to her notes. A mechanic looks down at his hands, up at a coworker or computer monitor, then back down to the objects he's manipulating. A quarterback rapidly converges and diverges his vision as he drops back, evades defenders, scans the receivers, and releases the ball. Police officers or firefighters run into buildings and have to focus quickly on objects moving through bright light and deep shadow, probably accompanied by sudden loud noises, and instantly make decisions about what is a need and what is a threat.

Converging and diverging our eyes, processing that information, and then acting on it is a complex task that requires precise coordination of a chain of muscles, organs, nervous systems, and processes within the body. The good news is that, with training and technology, we can strengthen those muscles and organs and teach ourselves to process inputs faster and more accurately.

CHAPTER 11
STRESS LOADING

I have good news. Because we are learning how to train the ANS and the body's response to actual and anticipated stressors, it's possible to prepare yourself better to wake up tomorrow and be better prepared to face what life will throw at you.

Stress isn't necessarily bad. Quite the opposite: stress is necessary because without it, our bodies would atrophy, and we would never grow or improve. Stress can make our muscles and minds stronger or weaker. It depends on the nature of the stress and how we respond to it.

Stress involves a cycle with three phases: a *stressor, stress,* and a *stress response*. A *stressor* is something, internal or external, that is trying to push our body out of homeostasis: hot weather, a flu virus, psychological fear, whatever. *Stress* is the condition and symptoms it creates: fighting to maintain 98.6, combating the virus, and anxiety behaviors. Our *stress response* is what we consciously or unconsciously do to fight that battle.

We can put stress cycles into one of two buckets, which we'll label *constructive* (that makes us stronger) and *destructive* (that makes us weaker). Consider training at the gym. Sally goes to the gym and deliberately introduces stressors (lifting weights, running the treadmill, etc.). Her muscles and cardiovascular systems become stressed by the increased load. She responds by following the program her trainer mapped out, drinking a protein shake, and getting a good night's sleep. The next day, she works opposite muscle groups. Sally's stress cycle is constructive because, over time, she gets stronger and faster. But it could just as easily go in the other direction. Bob goes to the gym but lifts too much weight for too many reps and runs too long without proper rest and recovery because he's anxious about an upcoming competition. Over time, he gets injuries and feels run down. He gets depressed, so he pushes harder, which leads to a downward spiral. Over a couple of months, Bob gets weaker and slower and starts feeling sick. So, Sally and Bob both went to the gym and worked out, but her stress cycle was constructive, while his was destructive.

In Chapter 2, we saw that the ANS always tries to preserve homeostasis. If the body is pushed out of its default parameters, the ANS will initiate protocols to pull it back.

We might think of these parameters as a range, what aerospace engineers call the operational "envelope" of an aircraft. A bigger, more elastic envelope means that the plane can safely execute a broader range of maneuvers and fly under more diverse conditions. In the same way, constructive stress cycles can make our operating envelope more elastic. We get stronger and faster, and our bodies can maintain homeostasis under a wider range of conditions. We stay healthy and safe even when facing adverse situations and environments. When a stressor hits us, we bounce back better. I call that dynamic resilience, and it makes us safer, healthier, and happier. But destructive stress cycles either shred our body's envelope so that we have no normal state or make our envelope so fragile that the slightest stressor can penetrate it, making us less safe, unhealthy, and unhappy.

We can try to control stress at each point in the cycle. We can try to limit the intensity or persistence of our exposure to the stressor (by walking away from it, for example). If that's beyond our control, we can limit the severity of the stress condition within our brains or bodies (by proper breathing or nutrition, for example). And, of course, we can adjust our response to the stress (with rest and recovery, for example). So, we can put spin on a stress cycle, sending it along constructive or destructive trajectories.

But stress cycles can have two other dimensions: *anticipatory* and *cumulative*.

What happens if your body anticipates a stressor that hasn't actually happened yet? Imagine standing on a boat, about to plunge into cold water. Your conscious mind alerts your unconscious ANS to prepare for a shock. Your ANS then proactively initiates some of these protocols: brainwave frequencies and patterns adjust, your heart rate and breathing accelerate, and your glands release hormones. Your body gets ready for the incoming stressor.

Or imagine living in a rustic cabin in the mountains. It's autumn, and you realize that winter is coming, so you start consciously storing firewood. But your unconscious ANS also tells your body to begin storing fat. So you feel hungry for the foods that can be converted easily to body fat, and the ANS switches your metabolism to start covering you in a warm, insulating layer of blubber. Your body is preparing to hibernate like a bear.

Or imagine being a combat soldier in a war zone. Night attacks keep you alert, so you sleep shallowly for short periods. Your brain hyper-focuses, flooding your bloodstream with adrenaline and cortisol to be ready for whatever might happen tonight. You don't know when you'll get your next meal, so your ANS tells you to eat as much as possible. Your metabolism converts and stores those calories, not as slow-burning blubber but as rapidly convertible sugars to fuel action on demand.

Those are examples of anticipatory stress cycles based on valid inputs: the water will be cold, the winter will be long, and the battle will be intense.

But what if the inputs are invalid? What if you believe something will be worse than it really will be, and your body prepares for the worst-case scenario? What if you're worried about losing your job, and your body responds by getting ready for cold, starvation, and incoming artillery? You'll start hyperventilating, overeating, and sleeping restlessly because you've exaggerated the anticipated stressor and triggered a disproportionate response.

Neuroscience, biology, and psychiatry are realizing that the causes and effects of stress cycles are far more complex than we realize. And because they are complex, these processes can become confused by faulty inputs and poor coordination, leading to dangerous conditions and fragile health.

The causes and effects are built around feedback loops. Eating pizza can be a protocol to lay in fat for a cold winter. Still, the metabolic changes it brings can also prompt you to lie on your sofa more often, watch even more TV, surf the web, and play video games for ten hours at a stretch. Which, in turn, affects your circadian rhythms and keeps you from dropping into deep, restorative sleep. Which then affects your memory and brainwave frequencies. Which then atrophies your cardio, respiratory, and muscular systems, bringing about hormonal imbalances and inflammations and weakening your immune system. Which then makes you want to lie around and eat even more pizza. Because the feedback loops in these cycles get overwhelmed, breaking out is challenging. You make a New Year's Resolution and buy an exercise bike or gym membership, but your body has redefined its default settings and sense of normal. You might make small changes, but they will have negligible effects until you reset the entire system.

And stress cycles become cumulative, which we call stress-loading. Sometimes stress becomes habitual. It could be thrust upon us by circumstances beyond our control, or we may accept or willingly embrace it because of our goals and cultural values.

Unpredictable, unrelenting, or unmanageable stressors can have nasty cumulative effects. An athlete might have pre-game jitters, but she knows when her matches will occur and can physically and mentally prepare for them. But an abused child who never knows when he will be screamed at or hit by an alcoholic parent lives with constant anticipatory stress. A struggling employee in a company going through hard times is constantly worried, trying to impress his boss and not lose his job. A single mother in financial distress can't solve the daily problems of child care, bills, and broken cars. All of these stressors can lead to chronic destructive stress cycles. The anticipatory stress forces the ANS to constantly reset its system defaults in preparation for the next crisis.

Chronic destructive stress cycles cause "stressed out" lifestyles. The stress load accumulates, and the consequences accumulate. Overeat for too long with too little exercise, and you'll probably get fat. Smoke or drink too much for too long, and you'll probably get cancer or liver failure. Sit around watching too much TV or playing video games for too long, and you'll probably have weak muscles and bones. If you suffer too much psychological stress for too long, your nervous system and memory will likely become unreliable. Do all of the above for too long, and you'll probably die younger and sicker than you otherwise would have.

This type of stress loading interferes with the ANS's ability to follow its prime directive of homeostasis. At a certain point, the body's concept of "normal" becomes warped, and its ability to rapidly or appropriately respond to change diminishes. The body becomes less resilient. We fall back into our chairs, unable to sleep well, focus, lose weight, or heal from illness or injury. Too much destructive stress for too long has taken too much toll.

So, what can we do about this? Can we fix the damage and adjust our stress cycles from now on?

Our medical industry's toolbox for "fixing" these problems is chemical intervention. Drug companies develop medications targeted to specific symptoms. And often, they work—or they appear to. They suppress the symptoms and thus create the perception of solving the problem. These chemicals are very good at temporarily shifting or moving the state of the ANS through something called "ligand-gated" (or chemically-gated) ion channels, in which a chemical such as a neurotransmitter binds to a particular protein in the neuron cell membrane and migrates inward. The response is rapid: the drug is administered, and the symptoms reside. As long as the chemical is present, the effect holds. But when the chemical is removed, the symptoms return. Thus, patients need their meds, or the behaviors (depression, anxiety, etc.) will return. They get stuck on medications without ever addressing the underlying causes. It's not worth getting too deep into the weeds here, but this is in contrast to something called "voltage-gated" ion channels in which the electrical currents of the nervous system can alter the state of neuron cells. For long-term changes in the function of the ANS, it's better to retrain the nervous system to regulate its electrical currents than to rely on neurotransmitter medications to treat symptoms.

It's not easy to fix past damage. If you have years or decades of stress load in your body, you must make significant changes to shed it. But the first step is to interrupt the process and get off the destructive stress-cycle train so that you don't add any more on top of what you already have. But how do you do that?

One way is to keep the ANS from kicking into its sympathetic fight-or-flight mode when there is no real-life threat. Unlike animals, the massive frontal lobes in our brains allow (tempt?) us to focus on abstractions and construct scenarios. We can imagine all sorts of "what-ifs" in the future or "what-abouts" in the past that trigger the same sympathetic responses as if we were being chased by a bear or trapped on a sinking ship. As we drive our car thinking about our job or lie in bed at night worrying about our 401k, we release massive amounts of adrenaline and cortisol into our bloodstream.

We exaggerate most of our anticipated stress. While some of us face physical dangers, most do not. To break these cycles, you need to mitigate your stressors or adjust how you anticipate them. Ideally, we'd do both, but most of us can't eliminate all of our external stressors. Life is full of situations, responsibilities, and circumstances beyond our control, and some stresses can't, or shouldn't, be avoided. You shouldn't avoid caring for children or aged parents, working to support yourself and your family, or serving your neighbors in need. But you can learn to manage your actual and anticipated stressors. And you can change your stress response to spin them along a constructive path to make you stronger. If you value your health, you should ask yourself what you can change. Have you taken on responsibilities or habits that cost you more than they are worth? Are your coping mechanisms exacerbating your stress, making it worse, and putting you into what could be a literal death spiral?

I have good news. Because we are learning how to train the ANS and the body's response to actual and anticipated stressors, it's possible to prepare yourself better to wake up tomorrow and be better prepared to face what life will throw at you.

CHAPTER 12
TRAINING AND TECHNOLOGY

If you really want to harden your ANS to be more dynamically resilient and aligned with your conscious will and goals, then you need a structured assessment and training program monitored by a coach using a complete set of diagnostic and therapeutic tools.

Throughout this book, we've been exploring how your mind-body connection defines your real-world performance and how that linkage is affected by your ANS. The ANS constantly shifts gears between sympathetic mode (fight or flight) and parasympathetic mode (rest and digest). These shifts trigger anticipatory and reactive adjustments in all your body's organs and systems. And in the last chapter, we learned that psychological "preemptive strikes" can sometimes override the ANS's prime directive of maintaining homeostasis. If our unconscious ANS is effectively balanced and efficiently operating with our conscious mind, we can harness mental and emotional focus, coherent power, and precise coordination. When it isn't, a cascade of biological responses can lead to performing below our potential or even stress-loading with adverse health effects.

What can you do to get and stay healthier and consistently perform at or near your potential?

It's tempting to look for shortcuts. Is there a pill? A surgery? An implant? A one-time treatment that will fix it? No, there is not. You can't reprogram your ANS by rewriting its internal coding. But you can indirectly train it to respond more to your conscious will. You can strengthen it to be less volatile and reactive to sudden changes and stresses. You can train your ANS like you can train your muscles to become stronger, your muscle memory to play the piano or swing a golf club, or your mind and tongue to speak a foreign language.

Just as with those types of training, you'll need to carry out defined exercises, over time, with real-time feedback to reinforce the right actions. If you do, you'll gradually gain more command and control of your body, and the mind-body link will become more reliable.

For decades, I've been training athletes, students, and business professionals using technology that measures the invisible processes in their bodies and gives them real-time feedback.

Biofeedback, EEG feedback, and vision training are technologies and therapies which electronically monitor autonomous, involuntary body functions so that your conscious mind can gain some measure of voluntary control over them. I say "some measure" because you will never achieve complete control, nor would you want to. These systems are built for your protection. Your ANS has fail-safes built into it so that you don't have to remember to breathe, digest your food, or tell your heart to beat. But you can learn to control these processes within a range of variability based on your inherent potential. And you can learn to keep them at the healthy end of that range, except in extreme emergencies.

In biofeedback, various sensors are placed on or around your body to monitor your heart, lungs, skin, and even your eyes and ears. Everything from your pulse rate, heart rate variability, respiration, sweat response, the salinity and conductivity of your sweat, the convergence and divergence of your eyes, and much more can be displayed in real-time on a computer screen in front of you. Using various training techniques, you learn to control some of these directly (i.e., breathing more deeply and slowly) and indirectly influence others (i.e., heart rate variability). Because you're watching the monitors, you can teach your conscious mind to induce specific involuntary responses. You learn what it feels like to slow down so that your ANS shifts into parasympathetic mode and how to initiate that shift with conscious thoughts and actions. Over time, your system becomes more responsive to these voluntary inputs and eventually finds new default settings. You teach your body to find a new normal.

EEG feedback follows the same principles but uses EEG technology. Small, noninvasive electrodes that read the electrical signals generated by the brain are placed at various positions on your skull. They measure the frequency and patterns of your brainwaves. In Chapter 7, we saw that these waves are classified by frequency (Alpha, Beta, Theta, SMR, etc.). The placement of these electrodes allows monitoring of different channels on the left, right, and center of your brain. Because the other regions of your brain control different functions in your body, EEG monitoring can tell us which wave frequencies dominate different functions and how hard the brain has to work to keep it all synchronized. With the electrodes in place, you can monitor what's happening in your head as you perform different tasks. And just like in biofeedback, you can recognize what sort of conscious thoughts and actions prompt changes in your brain activity. You can learn to calm down and focus because you learn what "calm and focused" feels like and how to summon it at will. You can learn what stress feels like and teach yourself to manage it.

Biofeedback vision training and EEG feedback can (and should) be combined with other health monitoring: sleep patterns, hormone levels, gut health, etc. But in reality, much of this is "downstream" of the ANS. Unhealthy hormonal levels are usually the result of some stress on the system, not their cause. But with wraparound data, looking at the body's systems from multiple vectors, we can form a pretty good understanding of what's happening inside you.

The process begins with establishing baseline metrics for all these factors. Then, based on variables like age, gender, general health history, etc., we can estimate your potential and establish goals for improvement. You may never have a professional athlete's cardiovascular system or a Nobel Prize winner's mental focus, but you can work to become the best possible version of yourself.

With your baseline established and your goals set, you can begin training and measuring progress. Just like strength training or learning Chinese, you can spend as much time and effort on training as your situation, goals, and resources allow. But over my decades of helping patients and clients train their autonomic nervous systems, I've learned that it is possible to make dramatic progress quickly. During the first few sessions, patients learn to recognize their sympathetic and parasympathetic modes and what thoughts and actions initiate them. Within a few months, they have significant measurable improvements over their baselines.

The same thing can be said for a lot of other skills. In a few months, you might learn to play songs on the guitar or have basic conversations in a foreign language. Those skills become part of your long-term memory. But for them to become deeply embedded in your "muscle memory" so they really become part of you takes continued practice and improvement. That's not to say that biofeedback vision training or EEG feedback therapy has to be continued forever. Still, it would be best if you continued exercising and developing the skills you learn in training to keep them from atrophying and to keep raising your thresholds.

Combined with accompanying therapies, biofeedback, vision, and EEG feedback training can help manage various brain-body issues. Anxiety and stress, of course, but also asthma, Attention-Deficit/Hyperactivity Disorder (ADHD), and chronic pain. It can manage the psycho-physical causes of Irritable Bowel Syndrome, constipation, and incontinence. Headaches, high blood pressure, tinnitus (ringing in the ears), and nervous tics all respond well to ANS training. You can work these noninvasive therapies into your schedule.

If you keep at it and continue to reinforce what you learn through this training, you'll gain more voluntary control over your body's involuntary processes and systems. You'll learn to recognize and manage stress effectively. You'll be in more command of your thoughts and have greater control of your actions. And you'll reduce the accumulated stress loads on your system that lead to many health problems and performance inhibitors that we can't seem to overcome.

How do you get started? There are an increasing number of self-training options. Smartwatches and other wearable technologies can measure your heart rate and give you breathing prompts. Smartphone apps can offer limited feedback and training suggestions for sleep and diet. These won't hurt you and can provide some general snapshots and prompts. But these consumer wearables are measuring effects that are downstream of the ANS. To understand what's happening upstream, causing these outcomes, we must measure and address the brain and nervous system. And these wearables and apps can't do that.

If you really want to harden your ANS to be more dynamically resilient and aligned with your conscious will and goals, then you need a structured assessment and training program monitored by a coach using a complete set of diagnostic and therapeutic tools. With that, you can begin forging your ANS into a suit of interior armor that can withstand stress and perform on demand.

CHAPTER 13
INNER ARMOR

Some of the time, energy, and resources that we spend now destroying our health will have to be reinvested in rebuilding it. And we will have to train ourselves to become stronger and more dynamically resilient. Only then will we live well, long, and perform at our true potential.

In many ways, modern people in developed nations are far healthier than they were a century ago. Antibiotics and vaccines have beaten back many of the diseases which have plagued humanity. Childbirth is safer, and infant mortality is lower than ever before. Surgical techniques and medical technologies have increased our ability to survive accidents, organ failure, and congenital disabilities. It ought to be a golden age of health for Americans.

But in other important ways, we are less healthy than our great-grandparents. We are heavier, and our bodies are under more psychological stress than ever.

We suffer from countless nervous, mental, and emotional disorders. Almost no one gets tuberculosis anymore, and smallpox is just a sad history lesson. Still, we have epidemics of depression, anxiety disorders, ADHD, diabetes, heart disease, respiratory failure, and even suicide...the list goes on and on. We're even getting sicker at a faster rate. Sixty years ago, polio was a real threat to our children. Today, one in three low-income male children is on stimulants for ADHD or antidepressants, and the percentage is snowballing. It seems that the more our technology evolves, the sicker we get.

Increasingly, we are becoming people that perform far below our potential. Children and students do less well in school, workers are less productive, and families struggle in all sorts of ways. We are experiencing a plague of stress-induced illnesses, drug abuse, and self-destructive lifestyles. Professional sports are the only areas in which performance keeps improving because the big money they generate encourages technology, training, and fierce competition. But I work with many pro athletes, and they all struggle to perform consistently at their potential.

How did this happen? How can all of the advantages and blessings of modern life have made us worse off? Perhaps our world is changing faster than we can adapt.

The ANS is constantly below the surface, responding to and anticipating stress by adjusting our organs and systems. Throughout most of our history, humanity lived in a world regulated by predictable environmental parameters: sunrise and sunset, a pace dictated by the speed of a human walking or a horse running, food grown locally and organically, and people mostly living together in intimate spaces. Light, noise, and stimulation rarely exceeded our capacity to adapt. Our ANS algorithms were finely tuned to keep us alive and healthy in that kind of world.

We need to pay more attention to how much technology has changed our lives and how the pace of that change is accelerating. During the Great Depression and World War II, the "Greatest Generation" listened to the radio. They saw movies by physically going to a theater. Not all Americans even had electricity in their homes. But even where there were electric lights, phonographs, and refrigerators, the daylight-dark cycle still regulated lifestyles. Your great-grandparents listened to vinyl records of Glenn Miller's *Moonlight Serenade* and *In the Mood,* and when it got dark outside, they began to think about going to bed.

The Baby Boomers were raised on television. But the TVs were small, in a big cabinet in the living room. They went to concerts and parties but called their friends to arrange their meetups on telephone receivers with twisty cords connecting them to the kitchen wall or from pay phone booths. They may have invented rock and roll, but they tuned in, turned on, and dropped out of an analog world. When they wanted to communicate in school secretly, they didn't text—they passed scraps of notebook paper. They played pinball and crude video games at an arcade, feeding quarters into the machine. They also grew up in a car culture, with suburbia spreading farther and farther out. Their parents commuted to work, they rode buses to school, and as teenagers, they drove to part-time jobs and dates.

The Boomers gave Generation X computers, 24-hour cable TV, and video game consoles. But the computers were big, crude, and slow. They could send some email messages, and early portals like Prodigy and America Online allowed them to check sports scores and news headlines but not much else. The games were addictive but not immersive. MTV played music videos, but Gen X had to sit in the den to watch them. But the lights were almost always on, the parents were often divorced or gone (they were the original "latchkey kids"), and they listened to music on their Walkman cassette players all day. They were becoming more disconnected from the natural or even urban environment, living increasingly inside a technological bubble of light, sound, noise, and distraction. Their parents drove farther to work, pushing them into structured sports and other activities to fill the void that family and church used to occupy. If they weren't playing video games or watching MTV, they drove through fast food places on the way to part-time jobs or after-school sports. Things were moving faster and faster.

Generation Y, the Millennials, can't remember when there wasn't an Internet. They grew up with 24/7 media and advertising. It saturated them, coming from multiple televisions around in their home, in immersive video games that were always on, even in their bedrooms, on the computer screens that became ubiquitous, on the digital signage at the mall, in their schools, on their cell phones. Their nervous systems have been boiled in a bright, noisy, digital sauce. Every second and every crevice of their lives is filled with motion, noise, light, and pressure. They never get off the digital grid. And their stress load (discussed in chapter 12) accumulates like credit card debt.

The next generation was locked out of school and is being raised on Zoom meetings and *TicTok* videos. It doesn't take much imagination to project the trajectory and effects of that lifestyle.

Hovering 50,000 feet over the landscape, looking for patterns, we can't help but notice that the emergence of 24/7 digital lifestyles corresponds with the decline of performance and the explosion of illness.

Coincidence is not causality. Yesterday morning, I sneezed, and then it rained in the afternoon. Those two events may have coincided, but they aren't necessarily connected. But the big picture suggests environmental and psychological stresses are degrading our autonomic nervous systems. Throughout most of human history, hyper-stimulation was a signal of danger—lightning, fire, war, attack from enemies or wild beasts—and our bodies reacted by fighting or fleeing. But our environments have changed faster than our ANS can rewrite its code. Our environment is tricking our bodies into thinking that we're in danger all the time, and our bodies respond precisely as they are supposed to. Our systems are stressed, never recovering or resetting.

Ironically, the same system in our body that protects us from stress is reacting by making us sick with stress-related illnesses. We have yet to evolve to survive in this new environment. But what are we supposed to do, short of moving off the grid to some mountain cabin or desert island?

We must work hard to strengthen our internal, involuntary systems to withstand the stresses of 21st-century life. There are holes in our armor that leave our organs vulnerable. We need to forge inner armor that allows us to manage these stresses and perform through them.

To do that, we're going to have to make changes. We're going to have to evaluate our lifestyle choices seriously. Some of the time, energy, and resources that we spend now destroying our health will have to be reinvested in rebuilding it. And we will have to train ourselves to become stronger and more dynamically resilient. Only then will we live well, long, and perform at our true potential.

My team and I at Inner Armor are ready to help you forge yours.

ABOUT THE AUTHORS

Dr. Timothy Royer (Psy.D., BCN, BCB-HRV), or "Doc" as he is known, is on a mission to change the world one brain at a time. That's why he co-founded Royer Neuroscience and Inner Armor.

Doc began his career as a pediatric psychologist in clinical inpatient hospitals. Over time, he became fascinated by how the brain operates upstream to influence behaviors and disease downstream in people's lives. He began experimenting with and developing technologies and methodologies to measure, train, and optimize the brain-body connection. His research has led to work with collegiate and professional athletes in the NFL, NBA, PGA, professional tennis, etc. At the time of publication, he has assessed or trained ten of the starting quarterbacks in the NFL. But he also coaches business executives, students, and ordinary people who want to learn to perform at their potential.

Doc and his wife live along the south Georgia coast. They are the proud parents of four amazing kids and one great dog.

Greg Smith is a researcher, writer, and media producer. Along with Doc Royer, he hosts the *Inner Armor Podcast*. He and his wife live in a pine forest on the coast of Lake Michigan with a golden retriever named Finnegan.

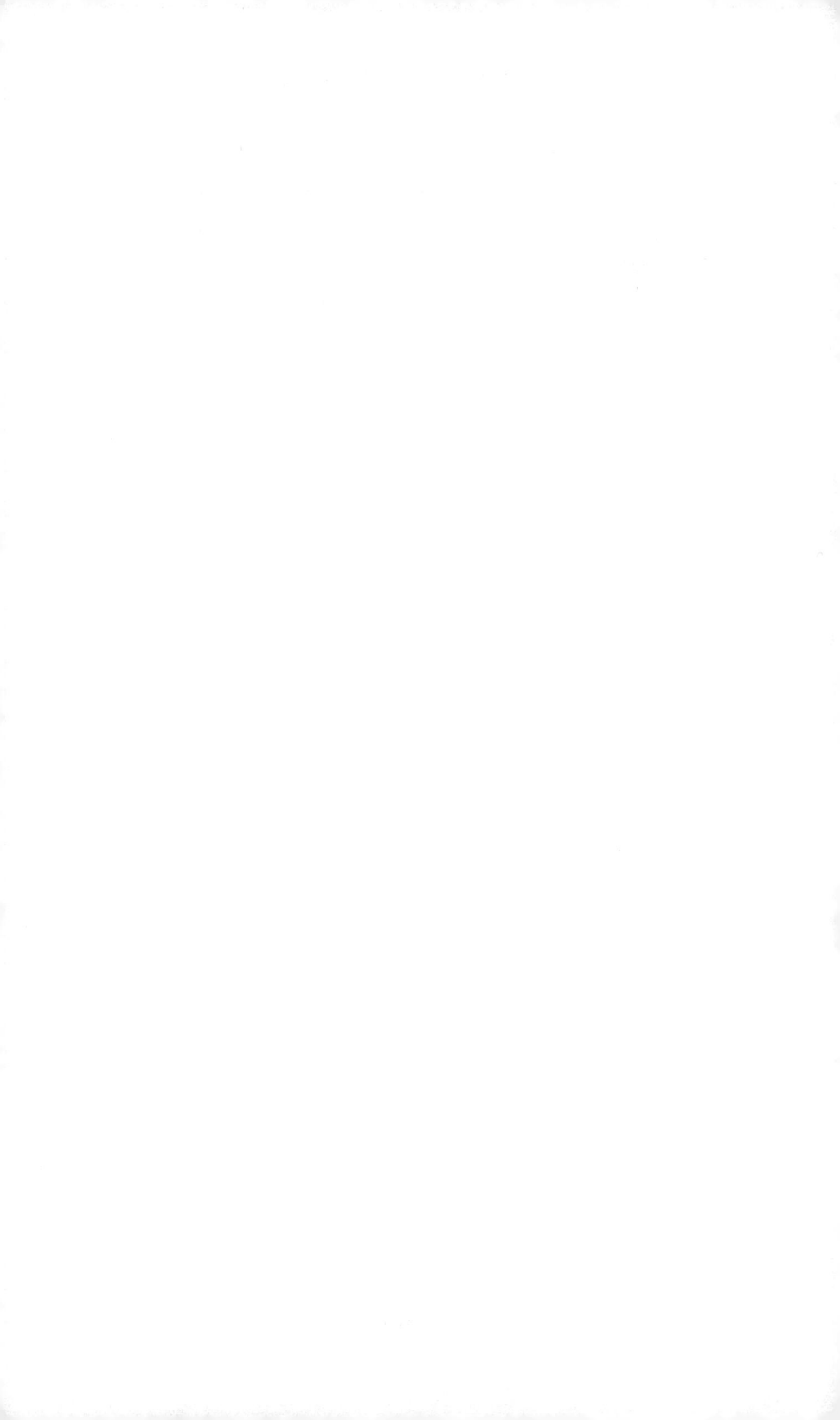

Made in the USA
Middletown, DE
29 March 2023